LOOK HOT, LIVE LONG

LOOK HOT, LIVE LONG

THE PRESCRIPTION FOR WOMEN WHO WANT TO LOOK THEIR BEST WHILE ENJOYING A LONG AND HEALTHY LIFE.

CHRISTINE LYDON, M.D.

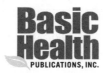

The information contained in this book is based upon the research and personal and professional experiences of the author. It is not intended as a substitute for consulting with your physician or other healthcare provider. Any attempt to diagnose and treat an illness should be done under the direction of a healthcare professional.

The publisher does not advocate the use of any particular healthcare protocol but believes the information in this book should be available to the public. The publisher and author are not responsible for any adverse effects or consequences resulting from the use of the suggestions, preparations, or procedures discussed in this book. Should the reader have any questions concerning the appropriateness of any procedures or preparation mentioned, the author and the publisher strongly suggest consulting a professional healthcare advisor.

IMPORTANT: If you have been diagnosed with or are currently undergoing treatment for any medical condition including pregnancy, please consult your healthcare provider before embarking on this or any other diet and exercise program.

Basic Health Publications, Inc.
28812 Top of the World Drive • Laguna Beach, CA 92651
949-715-7327 • www.basichealthpub.com

Library of Congress Cataloging-in-Publication Data

Lydon, Christine.
    Look hot, live long : the prescription for women who want to look their best, feel their best, and enjoy a long and healthy life / Christine Lydon.
    p. ; cm.
Includes bibliographical references and index.
    ISBN-13: 978-1-59120-024-6
    ISBN-10: 1-59120-024-5
  1. Women—Health and hygiene.
    [DNLM: 1. Nutrition—Popular Works. 2. Diet—Popular Works.
3. Exercise—Popular Works. 4. Movement—Popular Works. QU 145 L983L
2003] I. Title: Prescription for women who want to look their best,
feel their best, and enjoy a long and healthy life. II. Title.

    RA778.L96   2003
    613'.04244—dc21

                                                      2003001867

Copyright © 2003 Christine Lydon, M.D.

All rights reserved. No part of this publication may be reproduced, stored in a retrieval system, or transmitted, in any form or by any means, electronic, mechanical, photocopying, recording, or otherwise, without the prior written consent of the copyright owner.

Editor: Nancy Ringer • Typesetter: Gary A. Rosenberg • Cover: Mike Stromberg
Photographs: Randy Fauteux Photography • Illustrations: Karla Antonio

Printed in the United States of America

10   9   8   7   6   5   4   3   2

Contents

Part IV Appendices

Acknowledgments

To Bill Bush,
Thank you for your friendship and undying support. And thank you for putting me in contact with Basic Health; your intervention allowed me to write the book *I* wanted!

To Norman Goldfind and Nancy Ringer,
Thanks for your patience, your flexibility, and your talented guidance. Most of all, thank you for trusting my vision.

To Paul, Terry, Martin, Steve, Jason, Scott, Stewart, and all the rest of the gang at MuscleTech,
Your generosity and encouragement over the past three years made this book possible.

Wardrobe provided by LuluLemon Athletica.
Visit them at www.lululemon.com
2113 West 4th Avenue
Vancouver, BC V6K 1N6
Tel: 604-732-6111

Location provided by Kitsilano Workout.
Open 6:00 A.M. to midnight, seven days a week:
1923 West 4th Avenue
Vancouver, BC V6J 1M7
Tel: 604-734-3481

Introduction

Take a deep breath. This is not going to be as hard as you think. Contrary to popular belief, "eating right" is *not* synonymous with "deprivation and suffering." Likewise, "staying active" does *not* entail long hours devoted to a human hamster wheel. If that were the case, I sure wouldn't be able to pull it off. But even with a notoriously voracious appetite, an overflowing plate (literally and figuratively), and the attention span of a traffic light, I've always managed to develop diet and exercise strategies that enabled me to eat sizable portions of good-tasting foods while enjoying a lean, toned physique and excellent physical health. I wrote this book so you could do the same. *Look Hot, Live Long* is my magnum opus, representing the fruits of more than a decade and a half of medical training, health journalism, and direct involvement with the sports-fitness industry.

Working as a personal trainer, I discovered two distinct species of client. The first group surrendered completely to me through every aspect of diet and exercise. They put their trust in my expertise, rarely questioned anything, and proceeded through training with moderate success. In contrast to the first group, the second group questioned my methods, sometimes quoting books or articles that contradicted me. This group made real progress. And I learned something as well: People are far more likely to follow a prescribed eating plan or exercise program if they have a basic understanding of how and why the routine works to help them meet their particular training goals.

Hence, in writing *Look Hot, Live Long*, I have made every effort

1

to explain the logic behind my recommendations in reasonable detail. Many basic concepts recur throughout the book or are expanded gradually to provide an emerging awareness of the "big picture" of healthy living. At times, for the sake of completeness, I have included some rather involved scientific concepts. If you find the complexity of certain material too overwhelming to grasp in one sitting, skip over it. This information is not intended to confuse or frustrate, nor were these chapters designed to be memorized. If necessary, you can always come back to clarify elements that may have eluded you on the first pass.

At the end of each chapter (or subchapter), you will find a brief list of key points distilled from the chapter (or subchapter). These summations are included to reinforce important concepts and help facilitate positive lifestyle choices. For example:

REVIEW Key Points of the Introduction

1. Don't try to memorize the contents of this book; you can always refer back to specific topics.

2. Key points are listed at the end of chapters (or subchapters) to reinforce important concepts and help you implement specific lifestyle choices.

Live well, die old, and leave a beautiful corpse!

PART I

Good Nutrition Is Strong Medicine

Feed Your Nutrition IQ

Ironically, just about everything I know about nutrition I learned well after graduating from medical school. The sad truth of the matter is that traditional Western medical training tends to gloss over the concept of disease prevention and place inordinate emphasis on the concept of disease treatment. Unfortunately, many treatments offer little more than symptomatic relief and the promise of a protracted demise. Although this approach is far from optimal, it enables pharmaceutical corporations (which fund the vast majority of medical research performed in North America) to maintain a steady expansion of their multibillion-dollar industry.

Regardless of the politics behind this paradox, in the real world, the only completely reliable way to "cure" disease is to stop it from happening in the first place. Thanks to the growing influence of Eastern medical traditions (combined with the demands for better doctor-patient communication from Internet-savvy, surprisingly knowledgeable patients), the Western medical establishment has been obliged to shift gears. These days, many American medical students are exposed to the basic tenets of nutrition *before* they take the Hippocratic oath.

MACRONUTRIENTS

Macronutrients are the fundamental components of the foods we eat: carbohydrates, proteins, and fats. Let's start with a review of these basic macronutrients and the role they play in a healthy diet. Rest assured, you will not need an advanced degree in nutrition to grasp these concepts.

Carbohydrates

Carbohydrates contain 4 calories per gram and are the main source of energy for the body. Carbohydrates are subclassified according to their molecular size. A sugar that exists as a single 6-carbon sugar molecule is known as a monosaccharide. A pair of 6-carbon sugar molecules linked together is known as a disaccharide. Monosaccharides and disaccharides comprise "simple sugars." When three or more 6-carbon sugar molecules are joined, the resulting molecule is known as an oligosaccharide, or "complex carbohydrate." Complex carbohydrates are further subclassified as either starchy complex carbohydrates or fibrous complex carbohydrates. These various types of carbohydrates interact very differently with human physiology.

During the process of digestion, carbohydrates are broken down into smaller components and converted to the simple sugar known as glucose before they are able to enter the bloodstream. Most simple sugars you might ingest, including sucrose, dextrose, and glucose, are rapidly digested, rapidly absorbed, and rapidly assimilated. Their rate of entry into the bloodstream often surpasses the body's immediate need for fuel; those sugars that "spill over" wind up being stored in the body as fat. However, not all simple sugars are created equal: Fructose, the simple sugar found in fruit, is digested and absorbed very slowly. This is why it is virtually impossible to get fat on a high-fruit diet.

Unrefined complex carbohydrates tend to be digested and absorbed more slowly than simple sugars, providing a constant and sustained (though less intense) feeling of energy. Due to their slower rates of assimilation, the body uses unrefined carbohydrates as a longer-lasting fuel source. In essence, you can burn them at roughly the same rate as they enter the bloodstream, leaving little or nothing left over for fat storage. Whole-grain cereals and breads are good examples of slowly assimilated, energy-dense, starchy complex carbohydrates. Refined starchy complex carbohydrates such as white bread and white rice are another story. Like simple sugars, these foods tend to break down into glucose and rush into the bloodstream all at once, overwhelming the body's capacity to burn them as fuel. As a result, they are more likely to wind up stored as fat.

Foods composed primarily of fibrous complex carbohydrates include leafy green vegetables, broccoli, cauliflower, cucumbers, onions, peppers, and many other vegetables. In general, these food sources have high levels of moisture and insoluble fiber. Because insoluble fiber cannot be digested by the human GI (gastrointestinal) tract, it is passed as waste. Although adequate dietary fiber is paramount to a healthy colon, it is calorically vacant. Hence, foods classified as fibrous carbohydrates can be eaten all day, in enormous quantities, without causing any weight gain.

> **FIBROUS HEALTH**
> Although fiber is calorically vacant, it is, nevertheless, vital to good health. Inadequate dietary fiber can lead to a sluggish GI tract, water retention, bloating, constipation, and an increased risk of colon cancer.

Proteins

Proteins, which, like carbohydrates, contain four calories per gram, are the building blocks of living animal tissue. The structural integrity of virtually every part of the human body, including tendons, ligaments, muscles, and organs, relies on a protein framework. To maintain, rebuild, or add to existing muscle mass, the body must synthesize proteins.

Proteins are complex molecular chains composed of different combinations of twenty amino acids. The human body is able to manufacture twelve of these amino acids, but it lacks the enzymes necessary to synthesize the other eight. These eight amino acids, called *essential amino acids,* must be consumed in the diet. Protein-rich foods such as milk, cheese, eggs, poultry, red meat, and fish are rich sources of essential amino acids. They also are good sources of nitrogen, which is integral to protein synthesis.

During times of duress, such as surgery, illness, intensive training, or emotional upheaval, the body requires supplemental sources of three amino acids—arginine, glutamine, and histidine. These three amino acids are referred to as *conditionally essential.*

Proteins consumed in the diet are broken down by enzymes known as proteases, which are produced by the stomach, pancreas, and intestines. The proteins break down into individual amino acids or small "chains" of amino acids, called *peptides.* A dipeptide is composed of two amino acids and a tripeptide of three; anything larger is

The Essential Amino Acids

Isoleucine	Lysine	Phenylalanine	Tryptophan
Leucine	Methionine	Threonine	Valine

referred to as an oligopeptide. The individual amino acids and small peptides are absorbed into the bloodstream through the intestinal lining. Once in circulation, the amino acids are taken up by cells of various tissues, where they are either used to synthesize new proteins or are converted to glucose for energy.

The metabolism of amino acids is guided by the body's needs. When caloric and protein intake is adequate, amino acids are used for growth and maintenance of tissues, and the body is said to be in a state of positive nitrogen balance, a prerequisite for muscle growth. When caloric intake falls short of the body's requirements, amino acids undergo a process known as deamination, whereby their nitrogen group is removed, incorporated into urea, and excreted by the kidneys. The remainder of the molecule is converted to glucose and used as an energy source.

It is impossible to give adequate emphasis to the importance of adequate dietary protein, especially for athletes. Both strength and endurance athletes exist in a perpetual cycle of muscle deconstruction and reconstruction, and as a result, they have significantly greater protein requirements than nonathletes. Regardless of the sport, rigorous exercise results in micro-tears within muscle tissue. Contact sports and weight training lead to especially large degrees of muscular breakdown. Lacking sufficient protein intake, these tissues will neither develop fully nor recover rapidly.

Beyond the obvious aesthetic, athletic, and health benefits of maximizing muscle (lean tissue) retention, bear in mind that muscle is extremely metabolically active. Maintaining lean tissue necessitates enormous caloric expenditure even when you're just sitting around doing nothing. Adipose (fat) tissue, on the other hand, requires virtually no energy investment to survive. In essence, the more lean muscle tissue you possess, the more fat you will burn, regardless of your activity level.

Fats

American society has declared war against fat. Supermarket aisles are inundated with fat-free food alternatives. Exercise videos, too numerous to count, boast the latest fat-destroying workouts. A plethora of infomercials bear testimony to the mad proliferation of fat-burning exercise equipment. Even America's surgeons have joined the ranks. Employing techniques once reserved for malignant tumors, the great minds of modern medicine offer to permanently abolish offending fat deposits via surgical excision in the form of liposuction. It all seems to beg the question: Is lack of fat good for one's health? Should one's health be of concern when patriotism calls? After all, this is war . . .

At 9 calories per gram, fat contains more than twice the calories of proteins or carbohydrates. However, despite being such an energy-dense macronutrient, fat should not be eliminated from the diet. Far from it! The body needs fat for proper absorption of vital nutrients, oxygen transport, neurological health, cardiovascular health, reproductive health, skin and hair health, and proper immune function. Moreover, fat is absolutely vital to feeling sated or "full"; a small amount of healthy fat (derived from plant sources) should be included in every meal. In addition, fat actually retards the absorption of carbohydrates. Translation? When fats are consumed with a meal, they cause carbohydrates to be absorbed more gradually. Hence, your body has more time to burn glucose as it is produced, paradoxically decreasing the likelihood of fat gain.

MICRONUTRIENTS

Micronutrients comprise the vitamins, minerals, and trace elements necessary to good health. Because our bodies lack the ability to manufacture these vital substrates in quantities necessary for human health, they must be consumed in the diet. Although whole foods contain good supplies of vitamins and minerals, even a balanced, healthy diet may not provide adequate amounts for optimal health and well-being. Enter supplementation! But what exactly should you take, and how much should you take, and how often?

You are probably already familiar with all of the confusing acronyms devoted to micronutrients: RDA, USRDA, RDI . . . There's enough cryptic terminology to confuse Sherlock Holmes. In a nut-shell, the Recommended Dietary Allowance (RDA) for nutrients was first issued in the 1940s by the United States Food and Nutrition Board. The guidelines established by RDAs are updated periodically based on the latest scientific studies and offer different types of rec-ommendations depending on sex, age, and pregnancy. In the 1970s, the U.S. Food and Drug Administration (FDA) felt compelled to make the RDAs simpler and more accessible to facilitate food labeling. The FDA came up with its own U.S. Recommended Dietary Allowance (USRDA), which provides a single recommendation for each vitamin and mineral. Their recommendations generally correspond to the maximum RDA for each nutrient. To complicate matters further, the FDA has recently replaced the term USRDA with a new appellation, the Reference Daily Intake (RDI) (See Table 1 on page 11). But you probably won't find RDI listed on your multivitamin label. Instead, labels typically list the Daily Value (DV) for each nutrient. Expressed as a percentage, DV simply means the portion of the RDI contained in one serving of the product. Most multivitamins contain 100 per-cent of the DV of many important vitamins and minerals.

Should you take a daily vitamin supplement? The experts say yes. According to a recent article in *The Journal of the American Medical Association,* taking a simple daily multivitamin can significantly reduce your risk of developing a number of chronic ailments, includ-ing cardiovascular disease, cancer, and osteoporosis. However, many nutritional experts contend that the doses specified by the RDA and RDI—doses you're apt to find in your daily multivitamin tablet—may be adequate to suppress the overt symptoms of deficiency but not to prevent chronic illness or to promote optimal health. Which begs the question: Is taking a daily multivitamin enough to ensure that you're meeting your micronutrient requirements?

Unfortunately, there is no simple answer. A host of factors, in-cluding sex, age, diet, activity level, and general health, all play a role in an individual's nutritional requirements. Even occupation and locale can impact your supplementation needs. Hence, if your sup-plementation goal is to optimize your health and well-being rather than merely prevent illnesses associated with deficiencies, your spe-cific requirements probably exceed the RDI for many nutrients. Don't get me wrong—taking a daily multivitamin is a good place to start.

In the chapters that follow, you will find more detailed vitamin and mineral recommendations pertaining to specific health concerns.

Table 1. Reference Daily Intake		
Supplement	**RDI**	**General Action**
Biotin	300 mcg	Proper metabolism of macronutrients.
Folic Acid	400 mcg	Normal production of red blood cells.
		Normal manufacture of genetic material (DNA and RNA).
		Normal cell division and tissue growth, including fetal development.
		Reduces the risk of heart disease.
Vitamin A	5,000 IU	Normal vision.
		Normal reproductive function.
		Proper immune function.
Vitamin B₁ (thiamine)	1.5 mg	Proper carbohydrate metabolism.
		Nervous system health.
Vitamin B₂ (riboflavin)	1.7 mg	Proper metabolism of macronutrients.
Vitamin B₃ (niacin)	20 mg	Proper metabolism of macronutrients.
		Maintaining healthy cholesterol levels.
Vitamin B₅ (pantothenic acid)	10 mg	Proper metabolism of macronutrients.
Vitamin B₆ (pyridoxine)	2 mg	Proper metabolism of macronutrients.
		Normal hemoglobin production.
		Normal neurotransmitter production.
Vitamin B₁₂ (cyanocobalamin)	6 mcg	Proper metabolism of macronutrients.
		Normal red blood cell production.
		Nervous system health.
Vitamin C	60 mg	Proper immune function.
		Connective tissue health.
		Normal wound healing.
		Capillary health.
Vitamin D	400 IU	Proper absorption of calcium and phosphorus.
		Proper formation of teeth and bones.
		Normal insulin production.

Vitamin E	30 IU	Neutralization of cell-damaging free radicals.
		Cancer prevention.
		Prevention of premature aging and atherosclerosis.
Vitamin K	80 mcg	Normal blood clotting.
		Bone health.
Calcium	1,000 mg	Healthy teeth and bones.
		Normal blood clotting.
		Normal skeletal muscle contraction.
		Normal cardiac muscle function.
		Normal nerve conduction.
Chromium	20 mcg	Proper carbohydrate metabolism.
Iron	18 mg	Normal hemoglobin function.
		Normal myoglobin function.
		Prevention of anemia.
Magnesium	400 mg	Normal skeletal muscle relaxation.
		Healthy nerve conduction.
		Healthy teeth and bones.
Selenium	70 mcg	Prevention of heart disease.
		Cancer prevention.
		Cellular protection against toxins.
Zinc	15 mg	Proper immune function.
		Normal wound healing.
		Normal bone growth.
		Normal reproductive function.

REVIEW Nutrition Basics

1. Macronutrients are the fundamental components of the foods we eat and include proteins, carbohydrates, and fats.

2. Micronutrients comprise the vitamins, minerals, and trace elements necessary to good health.

3. Carbohydrates are energy-dense macronutrients that supply the body with fuel in the form of glucose.

4. Excess glucose that the body cannot use for fuel is stored as fat.

5. Consuming even large quantities of fibrous carbohydrates does not result in appreciable weight gain.

6. Proteins are the building blocks of human tissue and must be present in sufficient quantities for muscle toning to occur.

7. Muscle tissue is metabolically more active than adipose (fat) tissue.

8. Fat causes you to feel sated, and a small amount of healthy fat should be incorporated into every meal.

9. Fats cause carbohydrates to be absorbed more slowly, decreasing the likelihood of fat gain.

The Lean and Lovely Diet

S o, you want to drop some fat, fast. And you don't want to suffer in the process. In fact, you're sort of hoping that the mere desire to get lean will induce the transformation. This fantasy is no more far-fetched than many of the dieting sophisms that American women embrace as gospel. You know what I'm talking about— stuff like "just drink these two sugar-filled shakes and eat a 'sensible meal'" and you can use your fat pants to erect the terrace awning you've always dreamed of.

Well, thanks to our current understanding of human physiology and recent technological advances in food engineering, the simple desire to lose weight truly is just about all you need to actually get the job done. You do not need to go hungry. You do not need to survive on exotic beverages that taste like lawn clippings. And you do not need to spend any more time than you currently devote to cooking and food preparation.

In this chapter, I'll guide you through the basic concepts of lean eating, and you'll learn that there's a good reason a lean, toned body generally emanates health and vitality. Once you've got the hang of it, you'll realize that eating for a firm, toned physique is no more complicated, time-consuming, or expensive than just plain eating.

APPROPRIATE WEIGHT LOSS
Weight loss of one to one and a half pounds per week is considered optimal. Exceeding two pounds may place you at risk for metabolic slowing, muscle wasting, and rebound fat gain.

GLYCEMIC INDEX: THE KEY TO SMART CARB CONSUMPTION

The concept of a glycemic index involves a more detailed understanding of human physiology and hormonal interactions than you have encountered thus far. Not to worry! I have already lured you into understanding the basics of how the glycemic index of carbohydrates impacts energy utilization and fat storage. Now I'm simply attaching some fancy names to concepts you have already mastered. Why bother? Because it takes away the guesswork. By assigning a glycemic value to each carbohydrate source (see Appendix B), you can apply your current knowledge to a wide variety of common foods.

As we learned in Chapter 1, the sugar found in our blood exists in the form of glucose. The suffix "-glycemia" refers to blood sugar. Hypoglycemia, for example, is the state of having an abnormally low amount of glucose in the blood. Hyperglycemia, on the other hand, is the state of having an abnormally high amount of glucose in the blood. The _glycemic index_ of a food indicates the rise in blood sugar levels this particular food will induce over time. The glycemic index is directly related to the total amount of carbohydrates the food contains, as well as to the rate at which the food is digested into its component parts and absorbed through the intestinal walls and into the bloodstream. Typically, the more processed a food is, the higher its glycemic index is. High-glycemic-index (HGI) carbohydrates, such as sugary foods, rice cakes, and white bread, flood your system with glucose. The result, with which you are likely familiar, is an intense energy rush caused by transient hyperglycemia. Elevated blood sugar is unhealthy for your organs, and the body knows it. In response to hyperglycemia, the pancreas releases a large bolus of insulin, a hormone that rapidly clears glucose from your bloodstream. The insulin spike, as it's called, results in hypoglycemia, which can leave you feeling lethargic and hungry.

Glucose that is not used for immediate energy accumulates in muscle and liver tissue in the form of glycogen. Glycogen is the primary fuel source for muscle. It consists of a collection of glucose molecules that are chemically bonded to form a sort of lattice. When new glucose molecules become available for storage, they can be added to the lattice through the process known as _glycogenesis._ As glucose becomes needed to fuel various cellular reactions (like muscle fiber contractions), the pancreas releases glucagon, a hormone that signals the body to cleave simple sugars from the glycogen lattice through a process known as *glycogenolysis*. These simple sugars are then converted to glucose through a process known as *gluconeogenesis*.

Unfortunately for the dieter, the body's glycogen storage capacity is extremely limited. Any excess glucose molecules that "spill over" from our finite glycogen stores are converted to triglyceride molecules. Triglycerides are the fundamental component of adipose tissue (fat cells). However, unlike our muscle cells and their limited glycogen storage capcity, human fat cells have an enormous triglyceride storage capacity. We can store fat everywhere! Fat cells surround our internal organs and form a layer beneath our skin. Hence, fat can accumulate in a vast array of subcutaneous regions. Practically every part of our body, from our butt, hips and thighs to our arms, back and belly—even our face and neck—provides ample topography for fat deposition.

One way to minimize the process of fat deposition is to eschew high-glycemic-index (HGI) carbohydrates in favor of low-glycemic-index (LGI) carbohydrates. The lower the glycemic index of a given food, the more gradually it is broken down and absorbed from the GI tract into the bloodstream. Therefore, LGI foods induce a gradual insulin release from the pancreas, and the body has more time to use the glucose molecules for fuel rather than storing them as fat. Whole grains, legumes, most fruits, and yams all have relatively low glycemic indices.

Your weight-loss or weight-gain goals, activity level, and metabolic rate will have an important impact on the ideal type and amount of starchy carbohydrates you should include in your diet. Bear in mind that, as you make headway on your journey to look hot and live long, these parameters will probably evolve. Be flexible. As you become more active, gain muscle, and lose fat, your metabolic rate will increase. As your shape and conditioning improve, you will likely require more energy-dense carbohydrates to sustain your new body composition. Be prepared to modify your diet strategies to accommodate your revised requirements.

Carb Consumption for Weight Loss

If you have more than fifteen pounds to lose, I recommend consuming approximately 1 gram (or 4 calories) of predominantly LGI carbohydrates per pound of body weight per day.

If you find that you are losing in excess of two pounds per week, are sacrificing lean mass (as determined by body composition testing or by obvious muscle shrinkage), or are insufferably ravenous, add LGI carbohydrates to your diet in 0.25 gram increments every three days until you are losing no more than two pounds of body weight a week (or one pound every three days), you are no longer sacrificing lean tissue, and/or you do not feel overly hungry between meals. Sugar cravings do not count as hunger! They will dissipate on their own within three to six weeks.

Carb Consumption for Improved Body Composition

If you have less than 15 pounds to lose or you simply want to tone and firm without necessarily losing weight (bear in mind that muscle tissue weighs three times as much as adipose tissue), I recommend consuming approximately 1.5 grams (or 6 calories) of predominantly LGI carbohydrates per pound of body weight per day.

If you find that you are losing in excess of one and a half pounds per week, are sacrificing lean mass (as determined by body composition testing or by obvious muscle shrinkage), or are insufferably ravenous, add LGI carbohydrates to your diet in 0.25 gram increments every week until you are losing no more than one and a half pounds of body weight per week, you are no longer sacrificing lean tissue, and/or you do not feel overly hungry between meals.

If, on the other hand, you start to gain fat (as determined by

The HGI Fix

If you're trying to lose weight but absolutely *must* have your fix of HGI carbohydrates, restrict their consumption to breakfast and those meals immediately following cardiovascular activities. A good night's sleep or aerobic exercise depletes your muscles of glycogen. Your body uses carbohydrates consumed first thing in the morning or within an hour after a workout to replenish exhausted glycogen stores. In this glycogen-depleted state, it is unlikely that you will experience glucose spillover.

body composition testing), reduce your carbohydrate consumption by 0.25 gram increments each week until the fat gain has ceased.

> **BODY COMPOSITION TESTING**
> Most gyms employ fitness professionals who will gladly provide body composition measures.

Carb Consumption for Hard Gainers and Endurance Athletes

Are you one of those enviable individuals who can gorge like a wild animal and never gain an ounce? Do you spend hours at a time running, mountain biking, cycling, or swimming? If you have trouble keeping up your weight or if your exercise regimen includes aerobic sessions with durations in excess of 90 minutes three times a week or more, your energy requirements almost certainly exceed 1.5 grams of starchy carbohydrates per pound of body weight per day. Moreover, you will likely experience improved performance if you consume an HGI snack (such as an energy bar) just prior to or during your endurance training. (Don't count the HGI snack toward your total caloric intake.)

Start with a baseline intake of 2 grams of starchy carbs per pound of body weight per day, including an even mix of LGI and HGI index foods. If you find that you are losing in excess of one pound per week, are sacrificing lean mass (as determined by body composition testing), or are insufferably ravenous, add LGI and HGI carbohydrates to your diet in 0.25 gram increments every week until you are losing no more than one pound of body weight per week, you are no longer sacrificing lean tissue, and/or you do not feel overly hungry between meals.

If, on the other hand, you start to gain fat (as determined by body composition testing or visual inspection), reduce your carbohydrate consumption by 0.25 gram increments each week until the fat gain has ceased.

REVIEW Starchy Carbs in a Nutshell

1. High-glycemic-index (HGI) foods cause a rapid rise in blood sugar, which induces an insulin spike. This can result in hypoglycemia and hunger, not to mention glucose spillover and fat accumulation.

2. Low-glycemic-index (LGI) foods cause a gradual rise in blood sugar, which induces a gradual insulin release and gives the body more time to use incoming glucose as energy rather than storing it as fat.

3. If your primary goal is fat loss, start with a baseline starchy carbohydrate consumption of 1 gram of primarily LGI carbs per pound of body weight per day.

4. If your primary goal is improved body composition, start with a baseline starchy carbohydrate consumption of 1.5 grams of primarily LGI carbs per pound of body weight per day.

5. If you are a hard gainer or frequently participate in endurance activities, start with a baseline starchy carbohydrate consumption of 2 grams of an even mix of HGI and LGI carbs per pound of body weight per day.

BECOME PRO-PROTEIN

Most authorities now recommend that active individuals consume a minimum of 0.7 grams of protein per pound of body weight every day. If you are concerned about potential health risks associated with increased protein intake, rest assured: The medical literature reveals no evidence that normal, healthy individuals experience any unusual health problems on high-protein diets. In fact, high protein intake has been linked to both improved immune function and increased bone density. However, increased protein consumption should be accompanied by adequate fluid intake (at least two to four quarts a day), because the accompanying increased excretion of nitrogen wastes results in higher urine output.

How much protein do foods contain? As an example, each of the following contain about 20 grams of protein:

- 3 ounces of chicken breast
- 3 ounces of turkey breast
- ⅔ of a can of white meat tuna
- 6 large egg whites
- 2 ounces of lean beef
- 4 ounces of shrimp or lobster

For a more comprehensive listing, turn to Appendix A.

Unfortunately, merely consuming adequate amounts of protein is not enough. Because the body is unable to store excess protein, you must ingest protein every two to three hours to provide a constant supply of amino acids for lean tissue growth, maintenance, and repair. For example, a 130-pound woman would need to eat at least 91 grams of protein (130 x 0.7 = 91 grams). She might eat a breakfast including six egg whites (20 grams), followed by a midmorning meal of a 3-ounce chicken breast (20 + 20 = 40 grams), a lunch including two-thirds of a can of tuna (40 + 20 = 60 grams), 3 ounces of turkey cold cuts for an afternoon snack (60 + 20 = 80), and a dinner including 2 ounces of flank steak (80 + 20 = 100). If this sounds like a lot of work, I have good news. The latest generation of engineered foods makes meeting your protein needs simple, inexpensive, and convenient if you don't have the time to do so with whole foods alone.

If you're worried about getting fat by eating too much protein, take a lesson in human physiology and put your fears to rest. In order for ingested protein to be stored as fat, it must first be converted to glucose, a process that requires high levels of glucagon relative to insulin. This hormonal ratio occurs only when you are in the "starved" state, that is, you have not eaten for at least four or five hours. In order for your body then to convert the glucose to fat, high levels of insulin relative to glucagon must be present. This hormonal ratio occurs only when an individual is in the "fed" state. Because it is impossible for these opposite hormonal situations to coexist, your body cannot store excess protein calories as fat!

If you have not been consuming adequate protein up to this point, make a conscious effort to do so, starting now. I guarantee you will see and feel results within a couple of weeks. Your muscles will appear more toned. You will feel stronger. You will notice decreased muscle soreness after exercise and will feel more rested. You will probably observe a decrease in body fat and an increase in lean muscle mass. Maximize your potential: Only with adequate protein can you hope to reap the full benefits of your training program.

REVIEW Five Fabulous Reasons to Become Pro-Protein

1. Adequate dietary protein optimizes lean tissue development (muscle toning), which elevates metabolism and maximizes fat burning.

2. It is virtually impossible for your body to store excess protein calories as fat.

3. Adequate dietary protein enhances recovery and minimizes muscle soreness following exercise.

4. Adequate dietary protein bolsters immune function.

5. Adequate dietary protein helps prevent bone loss and osteoporosis.

USE FAT TO LOSE FAT

As you've learned, adequate dietary fat is crucial to both good health and weight loss. Fat helps prevent overeating by contributing to a feeling of fullness. In addition, because fat slows the absorption of glucose, it helps stabilize blood sugar levels while it reduces the likelihood that ingested carbohydrates will wind up stored as fat. Fat is also necessary to countless physiological processes.

A balanced diet should derive approximately 20 to 25 percent of its total caloric content from fat sources. However, as is the case with carbohydrates, not all fats are created equal. Understanding the differences among the various types of fat will enable you to direct your fat consumption to optimize both systemic health and—believe it or not—fat burning.

Saturated Fats

Saturated fats are usually solid at room temperature. Most animal products, including fatty cuts of red meat, egg yolks, chicken skin, cheese, butter, cream, and lard, as well as certain plant products like vegetable shortening, cocoa butter, palm oil, and coconut oil, are notoriously high in saturated fats. Consumption of saturated fats stimulates the release of insulin, which typically results in rapid storage of the saturated fats as body fat. Moreover, saturated fat intake has been linked to increased LDL (bad cholesterol) levels, cardiovascular disease, certain types of cancer, ischemic stroke, and diabetes. For optimal health, I recommend limiting saturated fat to 5 to 10 percent of your total daily caloric intake.

Mono- and Polyunsaturated Fats

Unsaturated fats are generally liquid at room temperature and solid when refrigerated. They include sesame, soy, corn, and sunflower oils as well as peanuts and peanut oils, olives and olive oils, almonds and almond butter, and avocados. Unsaturated fat consumption has been shown to raise HDL (good cholesterol) levels while simultaneously lowering LDL (bad cholesterol) levels. Unsaturated fats are also credited with reducing circulating triglycerides, which have been linked to an increased risk for cardiovascular disease, stroke, obesity, and diabetes. Use these oils in place of saturated fats whenever humanly possible.

A WORD OF WARNING

Avoid canola oil! Yes, it's an unsaturated fat. However, it is engineered from a plant source (rapeseed oil) that literally doubles as rat poison, and it has never been proven safe for human consumption.

Trans Fats

Through a manufacturing process known as hydrogenation, mono- and polyunsaturated fats are artificially "saturated" so that they will solidify at room temperature. The resulting products are called *trans fats.* Margarine is a prime example of a trans fat. Many manufacturers also add trans fats to vegetable oils to increase their shelf life. Don't be fooled by trans fats just because they come from an unsaturated source. Trans fats are even worse than saturated fats, for two reasons. First, manufacturers have brainwashed us into seeing these foods as "healthier" than saturated fats, and so we are less likely to use them sparingly. Second, a recent study published by the American Heart Association indicates that trans fats are significantly more damaging to the heart than saturated fats and have an even greater negative impact on cholesterol profiles.

Unfortunately, you may have a difficult time avoiding trans fats if you rely solely on nutritional labels. At present, manufacturers are not required to classify trans fats as such on the labels of their products. Until labeling improves, you can minimize your exposure to trans fats by using naturally occurring unhydrogenated oils (like olive oil) whenever possible. Likewise, choose soft margarine (spreads) over stick margarine, and avoid processed foods, fried foods, and snack foods like cookies and crackers.

Essential Fatty Acids (EFAs)

The essential fatty acids (EFAs) omega-3 and omega-6 are necessary for countless life-sustaining biological functions. Because the human body is unable to manufacture EFAs, they must be ingested from dietary sources. Both types of EFA are especially important for the dieter. Omega-3 and omega-6 EFAs not only aid in the prevention of muscle breakdown but also speed fat loss, raise HDL (good cholesterol) levels, lower LDL (bad cholesterol) and blood lipid levels, help maintain normal blood pressure, and act as natural anti-inflammatory agents. Their consumption has been linked to a reduced risk of cardiovascular disease, stroke, diabetes, and infertility. In fact, omega-3 EFAs are commonly prescribed as a supplement for relieving a wide array of pathological conditions, including glaucoma, depression, asthma, and numerous autoimmune disorders such as multiple sclerosis, rheumatoid arthritis, and lupus.

Omega-6 EFAs are found in many unsaturated vegetable oils and are abundant in most healthy diets. However, the average diet (even the average healthy diet) is completely deficient in omega-3 EFAs. To ensure that you are getting a full complement of omega-3s, try supplementing with two grams of flaxseed oil daily, and eat meals of cold-water fish twice weekly or take fish oil supplements (as directed on the label).

If your daily fare doesn't contain enough fat, add to your diet EFA-rich sources, such as flaxseed oil, walnuts, olive oil, avocado, and hemp oil. Avoid fried foods, fatty sauces and gravy, butter, margarine, and processed meats.

REVIEW Smart Heads Eat Fats!

1. Fat should comprise approximately 20 to 25 percent of your total daily caloric intake. Limit saturated fat to 5 to 10 percent of your total daily caloric intake.

2. Substitute unsaturated fats for saturated fats whenever possible.

3. Avoid products made with trans fats.

4. To ensure that you are getting adequate amounts of omega-3 EFAs, supplement with 2 grams of flaxseed oil daily and eat two cold-water fish meals per week or take fish oil supplements.

THE INFORMED CONSUMER'S GUIDE TO ENGINEERED PROTEINS

Recent engineering feats have provided the modern world with countless "timesaving" devices. Likewise, a combination of technology and entrepreneurial ingenuity has furnished us with numerous "timesaving" services. And let us not forget the "timesaving" shortcuts afforded by the communications revolution. But regardless of e-mail and mobile phones and shop-dot-com and pay-per-view and microwave ovens, time itself remains our most precious commodity. Ironically, any spare moments provided by technology tend to be devoured by technology's expanding possibilities. Women, in particular, seem to have an unusual penchant for heaping more and more tasks onto an already overflowing plate. Perhaps we are simply too hungry to experience all that has been denied us in the past.

From Olympic sports to world leadership to space exploration, the insurmountable gender barriers that confronted women as little as ten or fifteen years ago are gradually, and thankfully, dissolving. We have not simply joined the workforce, we *are* the workforce. While putting in at least as many hours as male counterparts, we still manage to tackle the lion's share of housework and child rearing. And through it all, we strive to stay active and maintain a healthy, toned physique. But given the demands of an already hectic schedule, who has the time to prepare six tasty, high-protein, low-fat, moderate-carbohydrate, nutritionally balanced meals every day? Nobody. The solution? Quality meal replacement in the form of engineered foods, such as sports bars and protein drinks. Which begs the question: What is it, exactly, that makes a particular engineered food a "quality" product?

First, the engineered foods you select should approximate the macronutrient profile (see "How to Calculate a Macronutrient Profile" on page 26) of the whole foods you would normally include in your diet. For most women, this equates to foods that are relatively low in carbohydrates and fat and contain a minimum of 20 to 25 grams of high-quality protein per serving. Which begs yet another question: What is it, exactly, that makes a particular engineered protein a "quality" protein? In a nutshell, the protein should support optimal lean tissue development. In order to do so, the protein must possess certain properties. For example, it needs to be highly digestible or it may never get from your gut to your bloodstream. As it enters your bloodstream, it must have easy access to target tissues—that is, muscle cells—or it may be diverted elsewhere. And once inside your muscle cells, it needs to contain all the necessary components to support new protein synthesis for lean tissue development and repair. In essence, a quality protein should possess properties of high digestibility, directed utilization, and optimal component profile.

Scientists have developed a number of different methods to assess

How to Calculate a Macronutrient Profile

The macronutrient profile of a given food is the caloric ratio of protein to carbohydrate to fat. It's relatively simple to figure out, provided you know approximately how many grams of each macronutrient are contained in the food item. For example, according to the nutrition information given on the package label, one Olafson's whole wheat tortilla contains 3.3 grams of protein, 18 grams of carbohydrate, and 3.3 grams of fat. We know that proteins and carbohydrates each contain 4 calories per gram and that fat contains 9 calories per gram. If we multiply the number of grams of each macronutrient by its corresponding per gram calorie content, we can determine the total number of calories of each macronutrient contained in the food item. In this example:

3.3 grams of protein x 4 calories per gram = 13.2 calories of protein

18 grams of carbohydrate x 4 calories per gram = 72 calories of carbohydrate

3.3 grams of fat x 9 calories per gram = 29.7 calories of fat

The total calories contained in the tortilla equals the sum of the calories contained in each macronutrient: **13 + 72 + 30 = 115 calories.**

If you now divide the caloric contribution of each macronutrient by the total number of calories, you will have the macronutrient profile of the tortilla expressed as a percentage.

13/115 = 11% protein

72/115 = 63% carbohydrate

30/115 = 26% fat

these properties and assign a "score" to various protein sources. Unfortunately, there is no one universally accepted method, and the controversy continues. For the sake of simplicity, I will employ the commonly used term *bioavailability* (BV) to refer collectively to a protein's digestibility, utilization, and component profile.

Let's spend a moment discussing component profile. In order to have high BV, a protein must possess a complete amino acid profile. If it contains insufficient quantities of a particular amino acid or acids (especially the essential amino acids), your body will encounter difficulties building the protein chains it needs. Think of it this way: If you had a magnetic refrigerator alphabet that included all twenty-six letters, you could spell anything, right? Wrong! Say you wanted to spell "momentous." M-O- . . . hmm, the M is already in use. What are you going to do now? If you were clever, you might take the W and turn it upside down to generate another M. Our bodies are pretty clever. Human physiology is capable of synthesizing all twelve nonessential amino acids from other amino acids. Problem solved! M-O-M-E-N-T- . . . uh oh, you already used the O, and there are no clever ways to manipulate the other letters to make an O. The O is analogous to the eight essential amino acids that the human body is unable to synthesize. Just as you could not spell the word "momentous" from the pool of available letters, your body can't arrange amino acids to build all the protein chains it needs when essential amino acids are in short supply.

Muscle is not the only part of your body made of protein. DNA, RNA, heme, hormones such as thyroxine and epinephrine, pigments such as melanin, and tens of thousands of other vital ingredients necessary to concoct a functioning human body are also made of protein. In fact, in the grand scheme of things, voluntary muscle is pretty low on the protein totem pole. In a crunch, your body isn't going to save its last precious amino acids to rebuild the muscle you tore apart during your leg workout. On the contrary, when the pool of readily available amino acids is lacking, the first thing sacrificed for the greater good is muscle tissue. Your body will gladly catabolize (break down) the protein comprising muscle tissue to provide amino acids for more important, life-sustaining endeavors, like manufacturing new red blood cells. Likewise, when glucose stores are dwindling, your body will catabolize protein to liberate individual amino acids, which are then deaminated (their nitrogen component is removed) and converted to glucose. Which brings us to another necessary component of any quality engineered protein: large concentrations of branched-chain amino acids (BCAAs).

BCAAs include the essential amino acids leucine, isoleucine, and valine; they are found in small chains or as free-form amino acids. Intramuscular protein breakdown begins with BCAAs, whose unique configuration facilitates deamination and conversion to glucose. Since one-third of muscle tissue is comprised of BCAAs, muscle catabolism is an unavoidable consequence of inadequate dietary protein and/or calories. In fact, up to 10 percent of calories consumed during exercise originate from the conversion of BCAAs to glucose. Studies demonstrate that BCAA supplementation not only enhances performance by improving endurance but also permits muscle sparing (the opposite of muscle catabolism) during intense training.

Now that you have a deeper understanding of what comprises "quality" protein, let's take a closer look at the most common sources of protein in engineered foods.

Egg

Once considered the "gold standard," egg protein now takes a backseat to many engineered supplements. To its credit, egg protein boasts a solid overall amino acid profile, and its BV is second only to whey. Unfortunately, egg falls short in comparison to the high concentrations of BCAAs found in whey and the high concentrations of glucogenic amino acids (amino acids that lend themselves readily to glucose production) found in casein. Lacking these vital attributes, egg protein derivatives are functionally inferior, especially for the athlete. In addition, egg protein is no longer the bargain protein source it once was. Not to mention one particularly obnoxious side effect to supplementing with egg protein derivatives: a shocking amount of smelly gas!

Soy

Soy protein powder is making a comeback. When it was first introduced, soy protein concentrate generally contained anywhere from 30 to 80 percent protein, but it had a poor amino acid profile and far too many carbohydrates per serving. In recent years, modern technology has equipped manufacturers with the ability to extract soy protein isolates. On the positive side, soy protein isolates are 90 percent protein and contain high concentrations of branched-chain amino acids, as well as the amino acids glutamine and arginine. Moreover, studies have shown that supplementing with soy protein may actually boost metabolic rate, decrease cholesterol and triglyceride levels, and help the body maintain lean tissue while dieting. Soy protein is also less expensive than quality egg or whey products. Unfortunately, soy protein contains limited concentrations of certain essential amino acids, resulting in poor BV. However, for those who abide by certain moral or spiritual beliefs that preclude the consumption of animal products, soy protein supplementation offers a viable (if not completely ideal) alternative to other sources of engineered protein. Soy protein products represent one of the few means by which vegans and lacto-ovo-vegetarians can consume adequate protein to promote lean tissue development.

Casein

Cow's milk contains about 6.25 percent protein, of which 20 percent is whey and 80 percent is casein. Casein has a glutamine (see "Training Supplements That Really Work" on page 133) concentration of 20.5 percent, greater than that of whey, soy, or egg protein. In addition, casein boasts a high proportion of glucogenic amino acids, which lend themselves to glucose production and help defer muscle catabolism during exercise. Casein also forms a gel that helps regulate the transit time of proteins in the gut, theoretically permitting time-released absorption. This property is believed to help prevent muscle catabolism during periods of fasting, such as when you sleep at night.

Despite casein's numerous selling points, the true test of its ability to promote lean tissue development lies in its BV. Unfortunately, casein's BV is relatively low, falling far short of every other major engineered protein source (plus most whole food sources) except soy.

Whey

Whey is one of the main byproducts of the dairy industry and is produced during cheese making and casein processing. Initially considered a waste product, whey is now recognized as a functional food with remarkable applications ranging from protein supplementation to immune support. Appropriately treated whey protein is essentially lactose-free, low in calories, virtually devoid of carbohydrates, and remarkably well absorbed from the human GI tract. Moreover, whey protein boasts an extremely high concentration of essential amino acids and the highest concentration of BCAAs (20 to 25 percent) of any single protein source.

But not all whey protein is created equal. Whey protein isolates (WPIs) represent the highest grade of whey protein. WPIs are more than 90 percent pure protein and less than 1 percent fat and lactose, and they have the highest BV of any known protein source. Raw whey or whey protein concentrates (WPCs) must undergo several complex refining techniques in order to yield WPIs. First, hydrolyzation chops the naturally occurring long chains of whey protein into short pieces, or whey peptides. Specific peptides are then extracted according to their molecular size and electronic charge via two additional techniques known as microfiltration and ionic exchange. These manufacturing processes are complex, delicate, and expensive. But they are the only way to ensure the production of true WPIs.

In addition to its unparalleled BV, whey has many functional health benefits, the most formidable being the role it plays in immune system support. Ten percent of whey's proteins are intact immunoglobulin antibodies, which may account for research findings demonstrating that dietary whey supplementation is highly effective at helping combat bacterial infections. Whey also has the ability to dramatically raise levels of glutathione, perhaps the most important water-soluble antioxidant found in the body. Glutathione is made from the amino acids cysteine, glutamic acid, and glycine. By rendering toxins inactive and facilitating their elimination from the body, glutathione protects cells against a variety of carcinogens, peroxides, and heavy metals. Glutathione is also intimately connected to immune system function and is necessary for lymphocytic (white blood cell) proliferation. Low levels of glutathione are typically observed in individuals suffering from AIDS, atherosclerosis, Alzheimer's disease, and cancer. There is a growing stockpile of research evidence demonstrating that including whey protein in the diet can significantly boost our ability to combat illness. Of particular importance to women, whey protein has been experimentally shown to stimulate the anabolic hormone insulinlike growth factor-1 (IGF-1), which is known to help prevent bone loss.

Casein versus Whey

The latest, hottest controversy raging among the protein pundits involves a heated battle between the whey proponents and the "protein blend" proponents. Champions of whey protein argue that WPIs boast unparalleled bioavailability and, therefore, support muscle growth and repair better than any other protein source. The protein blend advocates point out that casein, due to its slow transit time and gradual absorption, provides better muscle-sparing action than whey alone. They claim that you can have the best of both worlds by using an engineered supplement that contains both whey and casein. Who's right? In a sense, both arguments are correct. But my sentiments lie with the whey team. Here's why: WPIs are expensive to manufacture. Casein is cheap. Yet, when you compare the prices of the various engineered supplements, the blends are just as pricey as WPI products. In my honest opinion, adding casein to "improve" an engineered formulation is simply a thinly veiled marketing tactic to cut production costs.

What about the business of casein's delayed absorption, which is supposed to lead to decreased muscle catabolism? If you are eating the recommended five or six high-protein meals per day, you don't need to worry a whole lot about muscle catabolism. By consuming 20 to 30 grams of protein plus adequate carbohydrates and fat every two to three hours, you will enjoy stable blood sugar and energy levels while providing your muscles with a constant supply of amino acids for growth and repair. What about at night, during the fast of sleep? Let me make a radical suggestion: Be sure your last meal of the day contains whole food proteins. Whole foods, such as chicken, fish, beef, and eggs, have far greater BV (and superior amino acid profiles) than casein has. However, like casein, they are digested slowly, providing a gradual, sustained release of amino acids—the same "time-release" property that casein supporters tout as the latest, greatest miracle in lean tissue development.

REVIEW The Lowdown on Engineered Protein

1. Egg protein combines a high BV with a solid amino acid profile.

However, considering its low concentrations of branched-chain and glucogenic amino acids, egg protein is not the best choice for preventing muscle catabolism.

2. Soy protein contains high concentrations of branched-chain amino acids and glucogenic amino acids and boasts functional attributes that make it good for your heart. Unfortunately, its low BV makes it a poor choice for promoting lean tissue development.

3. Casein boasts a high proportion of glucogenic amino acids, and it forms a gel that permits time-released absorption. Both attributes help defer muscle catabolism. However, casein has a relatively low BV and is not the best choice for promoting lean tissue development.

4. What do I really think? Whey protein isolates, whey protein isolates, *whey protein isolates!* In terms of muscle sparing, lean tissue development, and functional attributes, you just can't beat whey protein isolates.

SOLVING THE MYSTERY OF SPORTS FOODS

Western civilization certainly does not lack in "sports" bars and drinks. They are readily available in an enormous variety of colors, flavors, and textures. Collectively, they boast an astonishing range of palatabilities, from mouthwatering to my-mouth-needs-water. Palatability aside, it's virtually impossible to find a more convenient and portable meal or snack. As you tear the technologically advanced wrapper from one of these neatly sealed units of contemporary nutriment, you can't help but sense an almost mystical melding of Willie Wonka and Neil Armstrong.

It should come as no surprise that the popularity of "sports" foods is growing at an unprecedented rate. Indeed, two decades of laboratory research have yielded bars and drinks purported to accomplish everything from enhancing muscular development and athletic performance to speeding recovery and fat loss to increasing your intelligence and/or virility. But do any of these space-age minimarvels actually live up to their marketing claims? Yes, some actually do. However, for every good-quality product on the market there are a dozen more that do more harm than good. As a consumer, you must be discerning to distinguish the gems.

> **CHECK THOSE LABELS!**
> Whether you are shopping for straight protein powder, ready-to-drink protein shakes, meal replacements, or high-protein/low-carb bars, if the first ingredient on the label is not protein, keep looking!

Energy Drinks and Bars

Endurance or energy bars and beverages have been around longer than any other category of sports food. Originally designed for long-distance runners, swimmers, and cyclists, energy bars and drinks are simply a high-carbohydrate, low-protein food source. With the burgeoning of fitness into a billion-dollar industry, energy product proponents (that is, the guys who make more money when more energy drinks and bars are sold) have done their damnedest to convince the average gym-goer that she too can benefit from their brand of sports nutrition. Don't be fooled. Endurance foods are for endurance athletes. Their general purpose is to provide immediate fuel for sustained aerobic metabolism and to replenish depleted glycogen stores during an endurance activity. The high carbohydrate content of the energy bar or drink is impractical for the average active woman who rarely engages in the extended-duration aerobic activities that would benefit from a high-carbohydrate meal. If you were to consume an endurance bar or drink prior to climbing onto the StairMaster for 45 minutes, the item's high-carb/low-protein content ensures you would burn very little fat during your cardio session. By the same token, after a cardio session, why would you opt to use an endurance bar to replenish depleted glycogen stores when there are any number of bars that, for the same price, would also serve as a significant source of protein? Remember, proteins, not carbohydrates, are the building blocks of a toned physique.

Meal Replacement Drinks and Bars

A meal replacement product is exactly what its name implies: a bar or drink intended to replace a meal with adequate quantities of macronutrients, vitamins, and minerals. In contrast to energy bars and drinks, quality meal replacement products contain adequate protein to constitute a healthy meal. The downside? Many meal replacement bars and drinks also contain high levels of carbohydrates, and if you are one of the millions striving to shed a significant amount of body fat, these high-carb meal replacements would be counterproductive to your goals.

Of course, at certain times a meal replacement bar is appropriate for replenishing glycogen stores and preventing muscle breakdown, such as first thing in the morning when we are in a "starved" state and our systems tend toward hypoglycemia or immediately following a training session when muscles are glycogen depleted. However, for the most part, unless you find a meal replacement product that closely approximates your chosen macronutrient profile, the excess carbohydrates may lead to glucose spillover and fat accumulation. When choosing a meal replacement product, insist on at least 20 to 25 grams of protein per serving.

High-Protein/Low-Carb Drinks and Bars

High-protein/low-carb products are ideal for promoting muscular development without concomitant fat gains. On the surface, a high-protein/low-carb product would seem to be the perfect snack solution for women on the go. Behind the promising facade, however, often lurks a taste so noxious it is offset only by the product's prohibitive cost. If an individual were both wealthy enough to afford the item in question and stalwart enough to choke it down, chances are good that said individual would be underwhelmed by the product's effectiveness. The unfortunate reality is that most high-protein/low-carb bars and drinks are made with marginal-quality protein that lacks sufficient bioavailability to impact lean tissue development.

If you're set on using a high-protein/low-carb product, select only those whose protein content comprises at least 40 to 50 percent of the product's total calories.

REVIEW Scoring a Goal with "Sports Foods"

1. If you don't honestly enjoy the taste of the engineered product, pass on it. There are good-tasting, quality powders, shakes and bars out there; don't settle for anything less.

2. When choosing a meal replacement product, insist on at least 20 to 25 grams of protein per serving.

3. When choosing a high-protein/low-carb product, insist that the protein content comprise at least 30 to 40 percent of the product's total calories.

TEN STEPS TO SHEDDING FAT FAST (WITHOUT EVEN TRYING)

I told you at the outset that this whole process of getting healthy and gorgeous would not be as difficult as you might think. So far, we've explored some fairly complex concepts. Here's a little breather: a handful of extremely simple routines that can help you shed unwanted fat with very little effort.

1. Know How Much You're Eating

Use this book or a similar guide to keep track of the calories, carbohydrate, protein, and fat content of your food. You should measure your portions (with a measuring cup or scale) until you have a good idea of exactly what one portion of a given food actually represents. Most people grossly overestimate portion size and hence grossly underestimate their caloric intake. Until your new eating regimen becomes second nature—a process that will take several weeks— you may find it helpful to record your eating and exercising habits in a diary.

2. Eat Frequent, Small Meals

Because eating temporarily boosts your metabolism, eating five 300-calorie meals is preferable to three 500-calorie meals. For the best results in terms of high energy level, diminished body fat, muscle growth, and good gastrointestinal health, eat five or six meals of 300 to 400 calories each day. Each meal should contain roughly the same amount of proteins and carbohydrates. Try to limit starchy carbs to the first three meals of the day and have only fibrous carbohydrates (fresh fruits and vegetables) with the last three meals of the day. To help ensure that you are eating the recommended five or six meals per day, make an effort to eat at specific times and places.

3. Drink Lots of Water

Water is vital to life, comprising about 70 percent of the human body. Water aids the liver and kidneys in detoxifying the body and eliminating wastes. The delicate balance of the body's electrolytes occurs in the water contained within and around the cells that make up all living tissue. Without sufficient water, we become dehydrated and our organs (especially our kidneys) cannot function optimally. Optimal kidney function leaves the liver free to do what it does best: turn calories stored as fat into calories used for energy.

Water is also an excellent diuretic. Not only will high fluid intake increase urination, it will also decrease overall water retention and bloat. Water also acts as a natural appetite suppressant. In fact, drinking water below your body temperature can actually help you lose weight. Did you know that consuming one gallon of water chilled to 4 degrees Fahrenheit will cause your body to liberate over 150 calories of energy?

Moreover, when you exercise, proper hydration leads to enhanced thermoregulation (body temperature regulation) and increased oxygen exchange in the lungs. Simply stated, the well-hydrated individual will have greater endurance and a more comfortable workout.

We do not feel thirsty until we are already in a dehydrated state, so it is best to drink water with sufficient frequency to prevent thirst. I recommend that every active woman drink a minimum of eight to twelve 10-ounce glasses of water throughout the day. So as not to shock your poor bladder, you may need to work up to this amount gradually over a week or so. Your reward for conscientious water intake will be clear skin, high energy, and, of course, fat loss.

4. Include Protein in Every Meal

Protein optimizes lean tissue (muscle) development, which elevates metabolism and maximizes fat burning. Moreover, excess protein calories cannot be converted to stored body fat.

Consume at least one serving (about 20 grams or 80 calories) of protein with each meal. Select lean protein sources, such as chicken breast, turkey breast, tuna, egg whites, and fat-free dairy products.

5. Emphasize Good Carbs

Derive your starchy carbs from unrefined, low-glycemic-index (LGI) sources like oatmeal, yams, whole-grain breads, lentils, and most fruit. Limit or, better yet, eliminate most high-glycemic-index (HGI) carbs like white bread, white rice, rice cakes, sugary sodas, corn flakes, and alcoholic beverages.

Enjoy plentiful amounts of foods rich in fibrous carbohydrates, such as leafy green vegetables, broccoli, cauliflower, cucumbers, legumes, onions, and peppers (see Appendix A for a more complete listing). Because fiber cannot be digested by the human GI tract, the vast majority of fibrous carbohydrates are passed as waste, without causing any weight gain. To ensure that you are consuming adequate fiber, I recommend including at least one serving of fresh fruit or vegetables with every meal.

6. Limit but Don't Eliminate Fats

Fat should comprise approximately 20 to 25 percent of your total daily caloric intake. Dipping below this ratio actually makes it increasingly difficult for your body to use fat as an energy source. In essence, your body "forgets" how to burn fat stores. Because fat causes you to feel sated for a longer period while stabilizing blood sugar levels, it should be consumed frequently, in small amounts, with every meal. If your daily fare doesn't contain enough fat and you find you must add fat to your diet, choose unsaturated fats derived from plant sources, such as flaxseed oil, walnuts, olive oil, avocado, and hemp oil.

7. Eat Breakfast

Give your metabolism a jump start in the morning with a healthy, high-protein meal. Breakfast will replenish depleted glycogen stores and keep your head clear, your energy up, and your concentration focused, even without coffee! No appetite in the morning? I have the perfect solution: How about a smoothie? Smoothies take only a moment to make, taste great, and are transportable. (See "Protein Smoothies" on page 39 for my favorite recipes.) What if you don't have even the five minutes you need to prepare a smoothie? Several leading supplement companies now manufacture ready-to-drink protein shakes. These shakes have great macronutrient profiles and can be stored anywhere you have a fridge available.

8. Eliminate Evil Enticement

Go through your cupboards and get rid of all the junk! If it's not there, you won't be tempted to eat it. Instead, stock up on fresh fruits, raw vegetables, and protein bars to be kept on hand for snacks.

9. Don't Drink to Excess!

Alcohol is the enemy of both good health and a lean physique. Ethanol contains 7 calories per gram, nearly twice the amount found in carbohydrates and protein, and is completely without nutritional value. Not only does alcohol contribute empty calories, it also slows the body's metabolic rate so that fewer calories are burned over time. Chronic drinking inhibits protein synthesis and muscle growth and repair, and it has a negative impact on the quality of your post-workout recovery. Acute alcohol consumption leads to a transient hypoglycemic state and subsequent food cravings. Finally, alcohol is hepatotoxic, so that even moderate drinking leads to fatty deposits on the liver. While the liver works hard to detoxify the system of alcohol, it is less efficient at lipolysis, or fat burning.

On the other hand, numerous studies seem to indicate that a drink or two a day may improve cardiovascular health. So, if you're going to drink, do so in moderation.

10. Slow Down and Use Positive Reinforcement

Don't inhale your food! Savor it. You will feel sated more quickly and, hence, consume less when you slow down, chew thoroughly, and take the time to enjoy your food. Realize that moderation is the key to long-term success.

Do reward yourself for progress. *Do not* punish yourself for setbacks. Speak of yourself positively. Imagine yourself eating well and exercising regularly. Use family, friends, and support groups as a source of encouragement and positive reinforcement.

If you can adhere to the above suggestions, you may *never* need to restrict your calorie intake again. Often, merely eating a healthy diet and engaging in regular exercise results in gradual, permanent fat loss, even without imposing any caloric limitations.

REVIEW Ten Easy Steps to Fat Loss

1. Know the nutritional content of the food you eat.

2. Eat frequent, small meals.

3. Drink eight to twelve 10-ounce glasses of water throughout the day.

4. Consume at least one serving (about 20 grams or 80 calories) of protein with each meal.

5. Derive starchy carbohydrates from LGI sources.

6. Be sure to include some fat with every meal; if necessary, supplement with fats derived from plant sources.

7. Eat breakfast.

8. Go through your cupboards and get rid of all junk food.

9. Avoid heavy alcohol consumption.

10. At mealtime, slow down, chew thoroughly, and enjoy your food.

PROTEIN SMOOTHIES

Protein smoothies are a quick, convenient way to boost your protein intake. They're also easy and fun to invent. Here are three of my favorite smoothie creations:

Protein Smoothies

EXTREME FRUIT EXPLOSION

PREPARATION TIME: 5 MINUTES • SERVINGS: 2

CALORIES PER SERVING: 324 • PROTEIN PER SERVING: 31 GRAMS • CARBOHYDRATES PER SERVING: 33 GRAMS
FAT PER SERVING: 6 GRAMS • MACRONUTRIENT PROFILE: 38% PROTEIN, 41% CARBOHYDRATE, 20% FAT

Ingredients	Calories	Protein	Carbs	Fat
2 scoops vanilla whey protein	220	40 g	6 g	3 g
6 tablespoons half-and-half	120	3 g	3 g	9 g
2 cups skim milk	160	18 g	24 g	0 g
½ cup frozen blueberries	60	0 g	15 g	0 g
½ cup frozen strawberries	37	0 g	6 g	0 g
½ medium frozen banana	50	0 g	12 g	0 g
TOTALS	647	61 g	66 g	12 g

Preparation

Blend the protein powder, half-and-half, and skim milk. Add the frozen fruit and blend until creamy. Hint: Peel the banana *before* you freeze it.

THE CAFFEINE ADDICT

PREPARATION TIME: 5 MINUTES • SERVINGS: 2

CALORIES PER SERVING: 215 • PROTEIN PER SERVING: 24 GRAMS • CARBOHYDRATES PER SERVING: 14 GRAMS
FAT PER SERVING: 6 GRAMS • MACRONUTRIENT PROFILE: 47% PROTEIN, 26% CARBOHYDRATE, 26% FAT

Ingredients	Calories	Protein	Carbs	Fat
2 scoops chocolate whey protein	220	40 g	6 g	3 g
1½ cups cold coffee	negligible	negligible	negligible	negligible
6 tablespoons half-and-half	120	3 g	3 g	9 g
½ cup skim milk	40	4.5 g	6 g	0 g
1½ cups ice	0	0 g	0 g	0 g
½ medium frozen banana	50	0 g	12 g	0 g
TOTALS	430	48 g	27 g	12 g

Preparation

Blend the protein powder, coffee, half-and-half, and milk. Add the ice and frozen banana, blending until smooth. Hint: Peel the banana *before* you freeze it.

BANANA COCONUT CREAM PIE

PREPARATION TIME: 5 MINUTES • SERVINGS: 2

CALORIES PER SERVING: 330 • PROTEIN PER SERVING: 34 GRAMS • CARBOHYDRATES PER SERVING: 25 GRAMS
FAT PER SERVING: 11 GRAMS • MACRONUTRIENT PROFILE: 41% PROTEIN, 30% CARBOHYDRATE, 28% FAT

Ingredients	Calories	Protein	Carbs	Fat
2 scoops vanilla whey protein	220	40 g	6 g	3 g
2 cups skim milk	16	20 g	20 g	0 g
¼ teaspoon almond extract	negligible	negligible	negligible	negligible
2 tablespoons peanut butter	180	8 g	7 g	15 g
⅛ cup coconut shavings	50	0 g	4 g	3 g
1½ cups ice	0	0 g	0 g	0 g
½ medium frozen banana	50	0 g	12 g	0 g
Totals	660	68 g	49 g	21 g

Preparation

Blend the protein powder, milk, and almond extract. Add the peanut butter and coconut and blend until smooth. Add the ice and frozen banana, blending until creamy. Hint: Peel the banana *before* you freeze it.

The Diet Survival Guide

Unless you reside in a dark cave with no access to television, newspapers, or e-mail, you are certainly well aware of America's obsession with dieting. This lambasting trend can be traced as far back as the 1930s, when women first became the targets of quack weight-loss schemes. These pioneering efforts, guaranteed to give a gal a gorgeous figure, have since proliferated into a $30-billion weight-loss industry. Much like their primitive counterparts, the vast majority of today's diet-related products, supplements, and books contradict the basic machinery of human physiology and, hence, are doomed to fail. More often than not, these so-called "diets" ultimately result in fat accumulation, muscle wasting, and ultimately, weight gain. Nevertheless, millions of us leap like brainwashed sheep every time a new gimmick comes along, certain that, unlike the other twelve fad diets we've already embraced without success, this one will work!

FAD DIET = BAD DIET

Numerous weight-loss plans have gained significant popularity in recent years thanks to extensive advertising and media exposure. Unfortunately, the vast majority of these diet schemes fail to withstand practical application or scientific scrutiny. Though many "fad diets" lure the dieter by encouraging her to eat as much of certain foods as she desires, they are actually dangerously restrictive, limiting caloric intake to starvation levels and omitting entire food groups and vital nutrients in the process. The restrictive nature of many of these eating regimens prevents the dieter from ingesting adequate nutrition for good health. Among the most common casualties of fad diets are important macronutrients like fiber, complex carbohydrates, and protein, as well as vital micronutrients including vitamins, minerals, essential fatty acids, and protective phytochemicals.

The take-home message? Fad diets can make you sick!

Although severe caloric restriction may lead to rapid weight loss, the very nature of such an approach precludes its long-term effectiveness. Weight loss that exceeds 2 pounds per week triggers hormonal modifications that our species evolved to survive times of famine. Metabolism slows. Fat retention increases. Muscle protein is catabolized for energy. Unfortunately, the loss of lean (muscle) tissue often results in a false sense of accomplishment. Initially, you do lose weight. However the "new you" is merely a smaller, flabbier version of the old you. As time goes by, the body does whatever it can to conserve its dwindling energy supply and prepare for more lean times ahead. Soon, weight loss grinds to a halt, and the dieter arrives at the dreaded weight "plateau," an impasse characterized by simultaneous protein breakdown and fat storage. Although body weight may remain constant for days or weeks, body composition deteriorates as fat accumulates and muscle is lost.

When the dieter eventually becomes frustrated with her lack of progress and terminates the diet, the weight rapidly returns—plus an added 10 pounds. Why? The muscle that was sacrificed during the period of forced starvation, combined with metabolic slowing, make it much harder to burn fat. In addition, the alterations in body composition (more fat, less muscle) ensure a lasting metabolic setback, and our dieter will find it even more difficult to shed unwanted pounds once she embarks on her next fad diet. Many people repeat this pattern over and over again, creating the vicious cycle of starvation and weight gain popularly referred to as "yo-yo dieting."

The take-home message? Fad diets can make you fat!

Once you know what to look for, you'll be able to quickly recognize the "fad" in a diet. For example, if a diet calls for a daily caloric intake of less than 1,200 calories, you are flirting with starvation and all its negative effects on body composition and metabolic rate. If the diet makes lofty claims or implies a weight reduction of more than one or two pounds per week, be wary. Remember, by preventing protein catabolism and concomitant metabolic deceleration, gradual weight loss helps ensure long-term success.

> **WATER WEIGHT**
> Much of the initial weight loss observed from dieting is simply water elimination. For the uninformed, this diuresis (increased urine output) can engender a false sense of accomplishment, encouraging the fad diet victim to continue her futile pursuit. Don't be fooled: Water weight can, and does, return.

There are other red flags to watch for. Fad diets often promote miracle foods, purported to melt your thighs while you eat. Please. The marketers of fad diets and fad diet products would also like you to believe that you can shed unwanted pounds without implementing lifestyle changes. As common sense would dictate, there are no magic bullets. There are no magic foods, special potions, or other sorceries that can single-handedly reverse the long-term effects of poor eating habits and lack of physical activity. Only with proper attention to diet, exercise, and supplementation can you achieve a lean, healthy physique.

For the sake of argument, let's take a closer look at some popular fad diets.

The Vegetable Soup Diet

All you need, according to this scientific breakthrough, is one head of cabbage, six large onions, two green peppers, one 28-ounce can of tomatoes, one bunch of celery, one packet of onion soup mix, and voila! You have the perfect food for a Third World prison camp.

Victims of the vegetable soup diet are encouraged to eat all the soup they want, plus paltry servings of fruit, brown rice, and potatoes. Dieters are wooed by the promise of up to 10 pounds of weight loss after only one week. Experts agree that vegetable soup diets promote water loss but not fat burning. Dieters can expect such pleasant side effects as gas, bloat, nausea, and light-headedness. You can probably guess at the source of the gas and nausea, but let me tell you a bit about the light-headedness. It is a cardinal symptom of hypoglycemia; in other words, when you're on the vegetable soup diet, there aren't enough glucose molecules floating around in your blood to fuel your brain. Between inadequate caloric intake and virtually no protein intake, your body is forced to catabolize lean tissue to meet the basic requirements for sustaining life. Wave goodbye to your hard-earned muscle.

The Fruit Juice Diet

The fruit juice diet is a veteran of fads. It first surfaced in the 1930s, and like an intrusive in-law, it just won't go away. Victims of this diet are permitted a handful of vegetables, tiny amounts of protein, and lots of citrus fruit. Proponents (that is, the marketers) claim that citrus fruit contains a special fat-burning enzyme. Opponents (that is, the scientists) assert that citrus fruit does nothing to actively burn fat.

Perhaps most alarming, the caloric intake dictated by the fruit juice diet is less than 900 calories a day—well below starvation levels. The combination of caloric inadequacy, nutritional vacancy, and lack of protein forecasts muscle wasting and extreme metabolic slowing.

The Food-Combining Diet

Supporters of the food-combining diet allege that combining certain foods while separating other foods results in thorough digestion, which, in turn, leads to weight loss. Apparently the creators of this wonder believe that millions of years of evolution failed to address the possibility that humans would eat a variety of foods in combinations dictated by availability. Proponents theorize that, without special food-combining practices, your digestive system creates "fatty buildups." I theorize that the proponents of the food-combining diet never passed high school biology.

On the first two days of this diet, corn on the cob, prunes, pineapple, iceberg lettuce, tomatoes, onions, strawberries, and baked potatoes are allowed (just the combination our prehistoric forefathers would have been likely to stumble across while foraging for sustenance). On day three, you get to gorge on grapes—just grapes. Although certain other foods are allowed during the thirty-five days of the diet, the choices are extremely limited. The lack of adequate protein and the elimination of food groups prescribed by the food-combining diet spell disaster in the form of muscle wasting and malnutrition.

High-Protein/Practically-No-Carb Diets

High-protein diets have recently gained formidable recognition. There is no doubt that a meal plan that emphasizes increased protein intake relative to carbohydrate consumption promotes fat loss and muscle gain, ultimately resulting in a leaner, healthier, and more aesthetic body composition. The dilemma lies in the fact that, when taken to the extreme, this diet (like many other "healthy" practices) becomes anything but healthy.

According to the American Dietetic Association, individuals who adhere to this sort of eating regimen are placing themselves at risk for long-term health problems. High-protein/practically-no-carb diets are high in cholesterol, saturated fat, and total fat, all factors that have been repeatedly shown to contribute to the development of heart disease, cancer, stroke, and depression. The diet is also low in fruits, vegetables, and whole grains, all of which have been repeatedly associated with a decreased incidence of these same conditions.

In addition, the prolonged carbohydrate deficiency called for by this diet results in an increased production of ketone bodies, which are derived from free fatty acids. Essentially, when "coming off" a diet that relies heavily on free fatty acid conversion to ketones, our metabolism behaves as if we have just survived a period of starvation. Hormonal modifications actually encourage fat storage in preparation for the threat of more lean times ahead. Moreover, the restrictions imposed by this eating regimen lead rapidly to boredom, at which point most dieters abandon the regimen and gain back all the weight they lost, plus some extra pounds for good measure.

Americans squander billions of dollars every year on weight loss, yet as a society, we are more obese than ever before. Although fad diets tend to camouflage their ludicrousness behind a veil of hokey "science," you don't need an advanced degree in gastrointestinal physiology or evolutionary biology to realize that fad diets don't work. As much as you might like to believe in magic, bear in mind, clever marketing does nothing to alter the laws of natural science. Indeed, the dangerous combination of caloric and nutritional restriction imposed by fad diets is actually counterproductive to weight loss. There are no short cuts. Healthy eating should not be viewed as a temporary inconvenience but, rather, as one aspect of a fit lifestyle that also includes regular exercise and intelligent supplementation. So, the next time someone tries to sell you on a miracle diet, tell them where to put their grapes.

REVIEW Four Ways to Spot a Fad Diet

1. The diet calls for a daily intake of less than 1,200 calories.

2. The diet implies a weight reduction of more than 2 pounds per week.

3. The diet promotes "miracle" foods purported to melt fat while you eat them.

4. The diet claims that you can permanently shed unwanted pounds without exercise.

SCALE DOWN ON WEIGH-INS

You've certainly heard of the rapid weight-loss schemes that promise you will "lose ten inches in one month!" What exactly are they referring to, anyway? Ten inches off your waist alone, or two inches off your waist, one off each thigh, two off your hips, an inch from each forearm, a half inch from each big toe . . . you get the point. The more body parts you keep track of, the more inches you appear to be losing. Does this mean that the concept of losing *weight* holds more validity than that of losing *inches*? Actually, no.

Many people who start exercising to lose fat find that they lose weight rapidly in the beginning and then seem to hit a plateau. If this happens to you, don't panic. Although you may not be losing weight, I bet you're still losing inches. Muscle is roughly three times as dense as fat. Hence, a given volume of lean tissue weighs roughly three times as much as the identical volume of adipose tissue. When you arrive at a point where you are adding muscle mass at roughly the same rate (pound for pound) as you are shedding fat, you will continue to lose inches even while your weight remains constant.

Don't be discouraged by a weight plateau. Because lean tissue is extremely metabolically active, the additional muscle you're building will ultimately help you lose fat. Muscle consumes calories even when you're just sitting around doing nothing. Adipose tissue, on the other hand, requires virtually no energy expenditure to survive. In essence, your muscle eats away at your fat! As you continue training, your muscles will eventually reach a steady state and you'll hit another plateau. If you're satisfied with the degree of strength and muscularity you've attained, your existing program should serve to maintain the muscle you've already built. Otherwise, you will need to increase the intensity of your training to continue muscle development. Long before you reach your training plateau, however, the rate at which your body is losing fat will probably overtake the rate at which it is gaining muscle and you'll lose more weight.

Be patient with yourself. Realistic, permanent weight loss takes time. As you learned in Chapter 2, weight loss of one to one and a half pounds per week is considered optimal. Exceeding two pounds may place you at risk for metabolic slowing and muscle wasting.

The take-home message? Whatever you do, *don't* worship your bathroom scale. Whether you're losing pounds or inches, diet and exercise will melt away the fat to reveal a new shapely you.

REVIEW Three Good Reasons to Toss Your Scale

1. Because a given volume of muscle weighs roughly three times as much as the identical volume of fat, fat loss is better judged in "inches" than in pounds.

2. Most people who start a diet and exercise program find that they lose weight rapidly in the beginning and then reach a plateau. However, although their weight may remain constant for several weeks, they are still losing fat and getting leaner.

3. Realistic, permanent weight loss takes time; exceeding two pounds of weight loss per week places you at risk for metabolic slowing and muscle wasting.

CREATIVE WAYS TO COMBAT CRAVINGS

The diet strategies we've discussed so far are not designed to leave you feeling hungry. On the contrary, healthy eating should have you feeling sated and energized. During the initial two to three weeks, you may experience mild carbohydrate cravings. Rest assured, as your body adjusts to the new routine, any cravings will diminish and eventually disappear.

In preparation for my first physique competition many years ago, I decided that for a period of eleven weeks I would eat nothing but skinless chicken breast, plain tuna fish, naked broccoli, and dry baked potatoes. Nine weeks into this misguided eating regimen, I went to the grocery store to restock my tuna fish supply. That's when I saw it—perched inconspicuously on the shelf of canned seafood like a diamond glittering amid a mountain of coal—an abandoned, half-eaten bag of M&M's. I glanced about furtively to see if anyone was looking, then I raised the vessel of delight to my eager lips and drank the pellets of pleasure as though my very existence depended upon their immediate ingestion. . . .

It's a challenge to remain true to a diet when ceaselessly faced with nefarious temptation. For most people, the word "diet" conjures images of deprivation and suffering. "Diet" is to "eat" as "budget" is to "spend," "prison" is to "domicile," and "lima bean" is to "chocolate." Nobody enjoys restriction. In fact, it's human nature to rebel against confinement of any sort. How, then, can we overcome our natural instinct to mutiny the ship of healthy eating? It's easier than you might think. After nearly ten years of lean eating, I've learned a few tricks that make the process far more palatable, literally and figuratively. To me, the word "diet" is no longer synonymous with tasteless, flavorless, endless woe. Read on to help make your voyage to a firm, toned physique nothing but smooth sailing!

Whet Your Wet

If you are not hugely fond of water (and I must admit I'm not), substitute caffeine-free, sugar-free, clear beverages. I have a supply of unsweetened herbal iced tea (Lemon Zinger is my current favorite) on hand at all times. Use four tea bags per every half gallon of hot water. Once the tea has brewed to the desired strength, simply discard the tea bags and chill the tea in the fridge. I also recommend sparkling water, both plain and with natural fruit flavorings added. For extra zing, add a teaspoon of frozen juice concentrate to a glass of your home-brewed iced tea (I recommend pink lemonade) or sparkling water (orange or grapefruit cocktail are my favorites).

Get Pickled

Kimchi, pickled ginger, pickled onions, and plain old pickles are all loaded with flavor and essentially void of calories. It actually takes more energy to chew these items than they return to the body in the form of usable calories. Theoretically, you could munch on pickled provisions all day long and lose weight with each bite. Bear in mind, however, that pickles are loaded with flavor largely because they are also loaded with sodium. Hence, if you don't want to expand like a sponge while packing in the pickles, it is absolutely imperative that you guzzle good old H_2O in copious quantities to prevent the puffiness that can result from increased sodium intake. (If you suffer from hypertension, please skip this particular trick.)

Feel Fuller with Fresh Fruit

You may be aware of dieting "experts" who recommend against fruit consumption for those who are trying to lose weight because of fruit's high sugar content. *Ignore them.* In contrast to other simple sugars like maltose, sucrose, and lactose, fruit sugar, or fructose, enters the bloodstream gradually and has an extremely low glycemic index. This explains fruit's uncanny ability to maintain energy levels during endurance activities. Fruits with the lowest glycemic indices include cherries, plums, grapefruits, apples, pears, grapes, and peaches. Fruits with the highest indices (which you may want to avoid or eat in combination with LGI foods) include bananas, papayas, and mangoes.

Moreover, because it's packed with fiber, most fruit boasts a high volume-to-calorie ratio. In other words, you can eat filling amounts of fruit without consuming astronomical quantities of calories. Pound for pound, melon is one of the most calorically vacant foods known to man. An entire medium-sized cantaloupe contains a mere 65 calories. A pound of watermelon? A trifling 50 calories. On the other hand, a small banana weighing only 6 ounces has around 100 calories.

I wholeheartedly recommend making fruit an integral part of your diet. In addition to being a valuable, natural source of antioxidants and fiber, fruit is a great way to maintain in-between-meal energy levels and stave off sugar cravings. On a more practical note, fruit is highly portable, readily available, and requires no preparation. If you love fruit, indulge!

One word of warning: dried fruit and fruit juice are another story.

Dehydration and juice extraction change fruit's volume-to-calorie ratio, resulting in a highly caloric and not necessarily filling snack. In the case of juice, little or no fiber remains. If you absolutely must have your morning glass of OJ, try diluting it with water or club soda.

Soup or Salad?

Begin your sit-down meals with a cup of soup and/or a small salad. The roughage in salad and the liquid in soup trigger the stretch receptors in your stomach, signaling your brain that you are starting to feel full. Not only does this little trick help curb your appetite during the main course, but it also forces you to eat more slowly. As a result, you will consume fewer calories over the course of the meal. Avoid creamy soups like clam chowder and broccoli and cheese soup. Instead, go for broth-based soups like miso and egg drop or other low-fat choices like tomato and split pea. Choose a light vinaigrette dressing for your salad.

Arm Yourself with Condiments

The old-school approach to weight loss advocated barren relics like severe caloric restriction, skipped meals, and lots of lettuce. The worst thing about being on a diet used to be that you were always famished. Nowadays, we're a lot smarter about eating for a lean physique. We know that by adopting a balanced, high-protein, moderate-carbohydrate, low-fat diet, we can effect fat loss and never feel hungry. Today, the biggest obstacle for dieters is the dread of bland, flavorless foods. Well, I'm just about the most untalented cook in the world, but I can tell you one thing for certain: You don't have to be a gourmet chef to make healthy foods taste interesting.

Condiments can make a world of difference. In my cupboard, at all times, you can find a supply of soya sauce, Parmesan cheese, ground peppercorns, mustard, garlic salt, hot sauce, and balsamic vinegar. All bland foods respond well to a little condiment coaching. For example, canned tuna livens right up with a little mustard or balsamic vinegar. Plain potatoes perk up with pepper and herbs. Skinless chicken breast tastes great with a splash of soya sauce or a dash of garlic salt. Plain rice or pasta is almost exciting with a sprinkling of Parmesan cheese. Even boring old egg whites take on new life with hot sauce on board. Condiments are your friends. Dare to experiment!

Be Naughty Once in a While

The high-protein/moderate-carb/low-fat diet you follow to burn fat may gradually lose effectiveness over time. As your body becomes accustomed to the routine, your metabolism is at risk for a gentle deceleration. A great way to combat this eventuality (while maintaining your sanity) is to plan to be naughty one day a week. On your scheduled "cheat day," indulge in meals that are higher in carbohydrates and fat. Satisfy some cravings. Eat pizza and chocolate! The abrupt shift shocks your system, forcing your metabolism into overdrive, and you will very likely burn even *more* fat on your cheat day than you would on a regular diet day. Moreover, knowing you have a cheat day to look forward to can really help keep you motivated during the rest of the week.

One word of caution: Don't go overboard. Limit your total cheat day consumption to between 500 and 700 extra calories worth of whatever you want.

REVIEW Seven Ways to Beat Your Cravings

1. Be patient! Most cravings will dissipate after three or four weeks of clean eating.

2. Add some zing to your water.

3. Snack on flavor-dense calorie-vacant foods like pickles.

4. Use fresh fruit to combat sweet cravings.

5. Start your sit-down meals with soup or salad.

6. Experiment with condiments.

7. Plan a weekly cheat day.

THE SKINNY ON FAT BURNERS

Combine modern society's lust for looks with our quest for good health and it should come as no surprise that health magazines, radio ads, TV news programs, and supplement companies have fueled the fat-fighting frenzy with an arsenal of lipid-pulverizing products. The modern consumer finds herself inundated with the claims of numerous agents touted as "fat burners." But which ones really work? It can be a daunting task to sift through the mountains of media hype and misinformation to emerge with a definitive answer.

As a physique model with a medical degree, I have a rather unique perspective on the supplement industry. My train runs at both ends of the tunnel. That is, my opinions are based on a combination of aesthetic principles and health concerns. The information I present in this chapter provides a blow-by-blow account of the reigning fat fighters you will find on today's market, including their proposed mechanisms of action, their safety and effectiveness as supported by scientific study, and their cost. I hope that the following evaluation will help clarify your understanding of current fat-burning aids to the extent that you will feel comfortable making an informed decision regarding your personal supplementation regimen.

Caffeine (Kola Nut, Guarana)

Caffeine, and its herbal equivalents, kola nut and guarana, causes a transient increase in circulating free fatty acids, which increases lipolysis (fat burning) and indirectly spares muscle glycogen. In addition, its stimulatory effects on metabolism make caffeine mildly thermogenic. Hence, caffeine consumption causes an incremental rise in the core body temperature, a reflection of increased heat production and caloric expenditure. Caffeine is a natural diuretic, helping eliminate subcutaneous water retention. Caffeine is also a performance enhancer; see Chapter 7 for more information.

For most, caffeine represents a safe, effective fat-burning, performance-enhancing substance. Despite much bad press, there is little to no conclusive evidence linking caffeine consumption to heart disease, cancer, birth defects, or even PMS. Be aware, though, that caffeine withdrawal is a very real phenomenon resulting in irritability, lethargy, and headaches. Moreover, caffeine inhibits the absorption of dietary calcium and could increase your risk of developing osteoporosis if your daily calcium intake falls short of 600 mg.

One final word of caution: Caffeine is passed in the breast milk and will cause agitation in the nursing infant. It should be avoided by pregnant and nursing women.

L-Carnitine

Carnitine is an amino acid that occurs naturally in several *isomers,* or molecular structures that contain the same kind and number of atoms but have them arranged differently. Unfortunately for us mammals, our bodies can use only the L isomer. Some manufacturers try to cut costs by selling carnitine products containing other carnitine isomers. Don't be fooled! Only the L form of carnitine is useful to the human body.

L-carnitine's theoretical ergogenic effects are mediated via two primary mechanisms. First, L-carnitine increases blood flow to skeletal muscle, which increases the availability of nutrient and fuel substrates while augmenting the clearance rate of metabolic waste products such as ammonia and lactic acid. Second, L-carnitine plays an important role in long-chain fatty acid transport into the mitochondria for greater beta-oxidation (a fancy term for fat burning), which results in glycogen sparing.

Though endurance studies have yielded mixed results, many sources advise L-carnitine supplementation for athletes because stores of this amino acid are rapidly depleted in the highly active individual. Recommended doses generally fall between 1 and 3 grams daily.

Chitosan

Chitosan is derived from the exoskeletons of ocean-dwelling crustaceans. One might wonder how on earth the consumption of seashells could possibly melt away unwanted pounds. As it turns out, several studies have demonstrated that chitosan may absorb dietary fat from within the small intestine. Because chitosan behaves as a fiber source and passes through the GI tract unchanged, it is eliminated as waste, along with any fat it's managed to engulf along the way. Sounds too good to be true! So what's the catch?

While research indicates that chitosan absorbs four to six times its weight in fat, manufacturers would like you to believe that a couple capsules of chitosan will enable you to quaff whatever you want, whenever you want, while your body magically transforms into an "after" picture. It just doesn't work like that. You'd have to take about 15 grams of chitosan to significantly impede absorption of the fat found in a couple slices of pizza. Also, chitosan is an equal-opportunity fat sucker; if you take quantities sufficient to impact lipid absorption, you can be sure you're also hindering the absorption of fat-soluble vitamins like A, D, E, and K, as well as the essential fatty acids your body needs for good health. Moreover, effective doses of chitosan have been known to cause stomach cramps, flatulence, diarrhea, and foul-smelling stools.

Chromium (Chromium Picolinate)

Chromium has been touted as the miracle fat burner: able to leap tall buildings and melt the cellulite magically off your thighs . . . While these claims may be far-fetched, the fact remains that chromium does play a central role in the metabolism of carbohydrates and fats, and chromium deficiency results in a number of untoward consequences.

Chromium is a necessary component of a hormonelike substance known as glucose tolerance factor (GTF). GTF enables insulin to bind to insulin receptor sites in the body, triggering insulin's physiological effects. Among its many functions, insulin facilitates glucose entry into cells for intracellular energy. It also promotes amino acid uptake by cells and stimulates protein synthesis. Inadequate dietary chromium can lead to increased fat storage, sugar cravings, fatigue, impaired athletic performance, suboptimal muscular development, mood swings, and poor memory. Long-term chromium deficiency is thought to contribute to cardiovascular disease, elevated LDL cholesterol levels, increased body fat, and the development of diabetes. Certain segments of the population have especially high chromium demands. These include athletes, pregnant and lactating women, and individuals suffering from diabetes or heart disease.

The best natural source of dietary chromium is brewer's yeast. Chromium can also be found in relatively high concentrations in the bran and germ portions of cereal grains. Unfortunately, due to the enormous proportion of frozen and processed foods that make up the American diet, as a nation we are notoriously deficient in this essential trace element. It is estimated that fully 90 percent of American adults are at least marginally chromium deficient. For active individuals, most references recommend chromium supplementation in the form of chromium picolinate or chromium niacinate to be consumed orally in the amount of 200 to 400 mcg twice daily.

Citrus Aurantium (Zhi Shi)

The immature dried fruit of the bitter orange, citrus aurantium has long been used in traditional Chinese medicine to treat congestion and indigestion and to promote circulation. Recent studies have demonstrated that citrus aurantium, or zhi shi, contains *adrenergic amines,* substances believed to mimic adrenaline in the central nervous system. Acting as a central nervous system stimulant, citrus aurantium is believed to raise metabolic activity and promote thermogenesis. For this reason, some manufacturers tout citrus aurantium as the "next ephedrine."

On the positive side, citrus aurantium does not appear to affect heart rate or blood pressure and could prove to produce significantly fewer adverse reactions than ephedrine-containing compounds. However, preliminary studies also indicate that citrus aurantium's effects are relatively mild, portending only a marginal increase in caloric expenditure through supplementation.

Ephedrine (Ephedra, Ma Huang)

Ephedrine is the active ingredient in many leading "fat burners" on today's market. It can be synthesized artificially in a laboratory or found naturally in flora of the genus *Ephedra.* The Chinese plant ma huang (*Ephedra sinica*) is only about 6 percent ephedrine by dry weight, though liquid ma huang extracts may contain far greater concentrations.

First used to treat asthma nearly 2,000 years ago, ephedra is classified as a sympathomimetic agent because it mimics the effects of the sympathetic nervous system. Ephedra works primarily through the release of excitatory chemicals called catecholamines. The catecholamines, which include adrenaline, act on cellular receptors found in numerous body tissues and are responsible for stimulating lipolysis, increasing heart rate, dilating bronchioles, decreasing appetite, and increasing alertness. Because it stimulates metabolic rate, ephedrine is said to be thermogenic, causing a rise in core body temperature and an increase in caloric expenditure.

On the negative side, ephedrine may cause nervousness, irritability, and hypertension in susceptible individuals. While ephedrine clearly has the capacity to be a useful adjunct to both performance-

enhancing and fat-burning regimens, it does demonstrate a low incidence of potentially dangerous side effects. My advice to everyone
who supplements with ephedrine and ephedrine-containing compounds is the following:

- ***Do not*** use ephedrine if you suffer from known cardiac abnormal-
  ities or hypertension or if you take MAO inhibitors.

- ***Do not*** supplement with ephedrine if you are pregnant or nursing.

- ***Do*** check with your health care provider before trying ephedrine if
  you have any other serious medical conditions.

Ephedrine, Caffeine, and Aspirin Stack (ECA Stack)

The most effective thermogenics contain a synergistic blend of
ephedrine, caffeine, and salicylic acid, or aspirin. When these three
compounds are combined, the desired effects tend to be more than
the sum of the whole. The combined effects of caffeine and ephedrine make for a powerful appetite suppressant, and their pooled
influences on metabolism increase overall thermogenesis, burning
more calories than either compound alone. Aspirin, or its herbal
equivalent, white willow bark, acts to prolong these effects by block-
ing the body's natural production of prostaglandins, hormones that
counteract thermogenesis by normalizing body temperature.

Numerous studies have examined the safety and efficacy of a
20-mg dose of ephedrine taken with 200 mg of caffeine. The trials
yielded excellent results in terms of safe, rapid weight loss. The general consensus throughout the scientific literature and the medical
community is that the components of the ECA stack, when taken as
directed by healthy individuals, are both safe and extremely effective
at promoting fat loss.

Guggul Lipids

Guggul lipids are derived from the gummy resin of the *Commiphora
mukul* tree, which is native to India. They have been used in Ayur-
vedic medicine for more than 2,500 years and currently represent
an effective, natural treatment for elevated cholesterol and serum
triglycerides. Various studies support the notion that guggul lipids
not only lower serum cholesterol, but also may reverse atheroscle-
rotic changes in vessel walls associated with elevated blood lipids

(hyperlipidemia). Under certain circumstances, guggul lipids have also been shown to stimulate gradual weight loss. Their proposed mechanism of action involves an increase in T4 thyroid hormone conversion to its more active T3 form. This conversion process normally takes place in the liver. Because T3 is about four times more biologically active than T4, increased levels of T3 relative to T4 cause a corresponding increase in metabolic rate and caloric expenditure. Unfortunately, studies indicate that the rise in circulating T3 levels may occur only in cases where the individual has suffered liver damage. In someone with normal hepatic function, guggul lipids may not have a significant effect, at least on fat burning.

Early studies using crude extracts of guggul lipids reported numerous adverse reactions, including diarrhea, anorexia, abdominal pain, and skin rash. Modern extracts are more purified and produce fewer side effects, though mild abdominal discomfort is not uncommon. Check with your doctor before administering guggul lipids if you suffer from liver disease, inflammatory bowel disease, or frequent diarrhea, or if you are pregnant or nursing. Also, be aware that many guggul products have undergone independent laboratory analysis and were found to contain few, if any, active ingredients. Seek out a reputed brand if you plan to try this supplement.

Hydroxycitric Acid

Hydroxycitric acid (HCA), the active ingredient in the fruit of *Garcinia cambogia,* has been clinically shown to inhibit ATP-citrate lysase, the enzyme responsible for the conversion of glucose to triglycerides. Because hydroxycitric acid suppresses the most crucial step in lipid formation, it helps prevent the storage of ingested carbohydrates in the form of fat.

Pyruvate (Calcium Pyruvate)

Pyruvate has been in the spotlight for the past couple of years or so, during which time it has enjoyed enormous media hype. Pyruvate is one of the end products of glycolysis, the process by which sugars and starches are metabolized in the human body. Of great interest to the athlete, pyruvate has been found to aid in the transport of glucose into muscle cells. Maximizing this transport process (known as glucose extraction) would theoretically increase endurance, fat loss, and muscle gain. In fact, current research indicates that the benefits of pyruvate supplementation range from enhanced performance to fat loss and muscle gain to reduced cholesterol and improved cardiac function. Unfortunately, the quantities of pyruvate found in food sources are inadequate to optimize its beneficial effects.

Until recently, manufacturers have found it difficult to produce a stable form of the substance. Now, pyruvic acid is combined with a calcium salt to yield calcium pyruvate, which is stable but not terribly affordable in quantities necessary to induce fat loss. Though most manufacturers recommend supplementing with 3 to 5 grams per day, test subjects needed to consume about six to ten times this amount—quantities which would be prohibitively expensive (not to mention inconvenient) to consume on a daily basis—to yield the desired changes in body composition.

With a modicum of dedication and consistency, you will actuate a physique to be proud of. While it's certainly tempting to try shortcuts, the hard truth is that fad diets and overnight weight-loss schemes don't work. The most effective approach to attaining and maintaining low body fat is to embrace a healthy lifestyle. Without proper attention to exercise and nutrition, all the fat-burning agents in the universe will not endow you with the lean, toned physique you strive to possess. However, by adding a proven, effective thermogenic to your fat-loss program, there is no doubt that you may significantly accelerate your results.

REVIEW Summary of Fat-Burning Agents

1. **Caffeine.** For most, caffeine is a safe, effective ergogenic aid with good fat-burning properties. Avoid caffeine if you are pregnant or nursing.

2. **L-Carnitine.** Most studies indicate that L-carnitine is a safe, effective ergogenic with good fat-burning potential.

3. **Chitosan.** Taken in large doses, chitosan may be useful for the chronically obese. It will not turn your four-pack into a six-pack.

4. **Chromium (chromium picolinate, chromium niacinate).** Chromium is an important trace mineral, especially for athletes. At

Beware: Fat-Free Foods Can Make You Fat!

The overwhelming propaganda in American culture advises us to strive for a fat-free diet. *Don't listen.* In fact, beware of "fat-free" foods. In many instances, it's actually healthier to eat the "fat-full" counterpart. Although a fat-full treat probably contains more calories than the fat-free variety, you're likely to gain more weight eating the fat-free variety. Why? Low-fat and fat-free snacks often rely on large amounts of sugar for flavor and texture. These sugars and refined carbohydrates rapidly enter the bloodstream in the form of glucose, inducing the pancreas to release insulin. Without the presence of fat or protein to retard the absorption of glucose, the resulting insulin spike will clear the bloodstream of glucose before you have a chance to burn it and it will be stored as (you guessed it!) *fat.* Because fat retards the rate at which carbohydrates are absorbed into the bloodstream, it functionally lowers glycemic index. Hence, a 200-calorie serving of regular ice cream will cause less of an insulin spike than a 200-calorie serving of fat-free ice cream, resulting in fewer calories stored as fat and a lesser chance of developing hypoglycemic sugar cravings.

Is eating fat free ever a good choice? Try the following rule of thumb: Fat-free foods are okay if at least 30 percent of their total calories are derived from protein (as is the case with skim milk, fat-free cheese, and fat-free hot dogs) or if you're ingesting significant amounts of protein with the fat-free item (as you might with fat-free mayo on tuna or fat-free cookies after a meal of chicken and veggies).

recommended dosages, it is safe for virtually every segment of the population.

5. **Citrus aurantium (zhi shi).** Citrus aurantium may represent a viable alternative for those who, for medical reasons, are unable to use ephedrine-containing compounds.

6. **Ephedrine (ephedra, ma huang).** Ephedrine is a highly effective ergogenic fat burner and potent appetite suppressant. If you suffer from a serious medical condition, check with your health care provider before using. Avoid ephedrine if you are pregnant or nursing.

7. **Guggul lipids.** Guggul lips are probably not very effective for fat burning, but they do hold enormous promise as a natural alternative for treating high cholesterol.

8. **Hydroxycitric acid.** Clinically shown to inhibit the enzyme responsible for the conversion of glucose to triglycerides, hydroxycitric acid helps prevent the storage of ingested carbohydrates in the form of fat.

9. **Pyruvate (calcium pyruvate).** The long-term side effects of high-dose pyruvate supplementation have not been studied. Try it (if you can afford it) at your own risk.

10. **Ephedrine, Caffeine, Aspirin Stack (ECA Stack).** In terms of thermogenesis and appetite suppression, you would be hard-pressed to improve on this stack. See caffeine and ephedrine (above) for medical contraindications.

Eat Your Way to a Ripe Old Age

During my first year of medical school, I remember being very frustrated with the overwhelming amount of seemingly unrelated facts that I was expected to memorize. But as the semesters rolled by, I realized there was a thread of commonality to the endless supply of details. Basic principles introduced during biochemistry were later reinforced by subjects like physiology and pharmacology. The excruciating minutia of human anatomy and embryology finally gelled during surgical rotations. In the end, the study of medicine turned out to be not so much rote memorization as recognizing common patterns and applying these fundamentals to a wide array of systems.

What I'm trying to say in my roundabout way is *don't* be intimidated by the number of discrete dietary categories that follow. Eating for a healthy heart is no more complex or time-consuming than eating to promote gut health, mental health, or bone health. As will soon become apparent, many aspects of these "separate" diet strategies overlap to a tremendous extent. By eating to strengthen any one particular system, it is virtually impossible *not* to beneficially affect all aspects of your health.

FOODS FOR A HEALTHY HEART AND VESSELS

The average total serum cholesterol for people of Western nations is 210 mg/dl (milligrams per deciliter). This statistic portends a 50 percent mortality rate from stroke and heart attack resulting from cardiovascular disease. Individuals with levels below 180 mg/dl rarely suffer from cardiovascular disease. In fact, according to the widely publicized Framingham study, the presence of cardiovascular disease is virtually unknown at cholesterol levels below 150 mg/dl. The bottom line: Every 1 percent drop in total serum cholesterol translates to a 2.5 percent decrease in the risk of premature death from cardiovascular disease. How can we capitalize on this fact to improve our foreboding predicament? In a nutshell, we can eat less saturated fat and cholesterol (from animal sources) and more omega-3 fatty acids (from plants and fish). We can lose weight and stay active. We can quit smoking. And we can take a lesson from the humble soy bean.

The fact that many Third World and Asian populations enjoy significantly lower serum cholesterol levels than we do relates directly to the large amounts of soy protein in their diet. Soy protein contains an abundance of isoflavones and other plant sterols, natural derivatives that mimic healthy hormonal activity. Research has shown that, over time, the regular consumption of isoflavones can reduce both serum cholesterol and triglyceride levels in human subjects. In fact, the daily consumption of 25 grams of soy protein can result in a 10 percent reduction in total serum cholesterol. And that's just the tip of the iceberg. A growing number of so-called "functional foods," which boast health-enhancing properties beyond their nutritional values, will soon be making their way to a supermarket near you. Be on the lookout for margarine derived from plant sterols that have been shown to lower total serum cholesterol by up to 10 percent, and keep your eyes peeled for new fiber-enriched products like pasta, frozen entrees, bread, cereal, chips, and even cookies.

Regardless of the latest and greatest in nutrition science, let's not overlook the established cornerstones of healthy eating . . . Fruit and vegetable lovers, lend me your ears!

Eighty percent of strokes and other cerebrovascular "accidents" occur because arteries feeding the brain become blocked by fatty deposits or blood clots. When the brain is deprived of blood and oxygen, even for a very short period of time, debilitating cognitive injury, paralysis, muscle weakness, aphasia (speaking and language difficulties), and even death can result. According to research, individuals who consume at least five servings of fruits and vegetables each day are about one-third less likely to suffer a stroke than those who do not. If you eat large quantities of broccoli, cabbage, cauliflower, and Brussels sprouts, and/or fruits which contain high concentrations of vitamin C, including citrus fruits and juices, your stroke risk is reduced even further.

REVIEW Five Cutting-Edge Steps to Vascular Health

1. Eat a diet low in saturated fat and cholesterol. Emphasize fruits, vegetables, soy products, low-fat dairy products, whole grains, and lean cuts of meat, fish, or poultry.

2. Consume an abundance of omega-3 polyunsaturated fatty acids. This "good" fat occurs in high concentrations in fish. In fact, the American Heart Association recommends three fish meals each week.

3. Maintain a healthy body weight.

4. Exercise regularly.

5. Don't smoke.

BONE BITES

In the United States alone, an excess of $15 billion is spent annually to treat fractures in people over the age of sixty-five. According to current research, a straightforward solution to this costly and potentially life-threatening problem includes daily supplementation with calcium and vitamin D, a simple regimen that can prevent more than half of broken bones suffered by seniors. In a nutshell, adequate calcium intake is essential for establishing and maintaining high bone density, and vitamin D is necessary for proper calcium absorption and utilization. Millions of men and women worldwide who either exhibit osteoporotic symptoms or are at high risk could benefit from consuming 1,200 mg of calcium per day, including dietary calcium sources, in addition to 400 IU of vitamin D.

The saturation of specific sites on the bone protein known as osteocalcin has been directly linked to bone strength. Epidemiological evidence also indicates that vitamin K, administered at roughly four times the USRDA, improves both osteocalcin saturation and overall bone health.

Vitamin C, or ascorbic acid, is one of the eight essential vitamins. Unlike most mammals, humans lack the enzymes necessary to manufacture vitamin C from its components and must, instead, consume it in diet. Vitamin C is essential to the manufacture of collagen, the main protein substance of the human body. Epidemiological studies report a positive correlation between vitamin C intake and bone density. For optimal bone health, I recommend supplementing with 500 mg of vitamin C twice daily.

What about protein? It is a popular misconception that a high-protein diet results in calcium wasting (excess calcium being excreted in the urine) and, consequently, may increase an individual's propensity to develop osteoporosis. However, cutting-edge research indicates that the naturally occurring phosphorus found in protein-rich whole foods actually prevents the loss of calcium from the body. Since virtually all protein sources (such as meat, fish, eggs, poultry, and dairy-based supplements such as whey) contain adequate phosphorus to protect against urinary calcium wasting, women and seniors should *not* limit their intake of protein-rich foods for fear of developing osteoporosis. In fact, low serum protein (protein found in the blood) has been linked to increased incidence of hip fractures in the elderly.

Supplementation aside, the best method for maintaining and even restoring bone density is to engage in regular, moderate weight-bearing exercise. This can include walking, running, and/or resistance training.

REVIEW Five Surefire Ways to Build Your Bones

1. Supplement with 500 to 750 mg of calcium twice daily.

2. Supplement with 400 IU of vitamin D daily.

3. Aim for a daily vitamin K intake (whole food sources plus supplementation) of at least 250 mcg.

4. Supplement with 500 mg of vitamin C twice daily.

5. Engage in regular, moderate weight-bearing exercise.

GRUB FOR GUT HEALTH

In order to reap the benefits of a balanced, healthy diet, your gastrointestinal (GI) tract must be capable of properly digesting and absorbing a vast assemblage of macronutrients and micronutrients. Think of it this way: If your body was an apartment building, your

GI tract would be the doorman. A competent doorman would permit entry to the tenants who reside in the building as well as the maintenance workers and delivery people who service it. An incompetent doorman, on the other hand, might refuse entry to authorized individuals. Worse yet, he might doze off at his post, allowing burglars and vandals to gain entry. Similarly, if your GI tract isn't functioning at peak efficiency, it might fail to absorb vital nutrients while allowing harmful substances like toxins and pathogens to pass directly into your bloodstream. Don't let a faulty GI tract sabotage your commitment to a healthy lifestyle!

The Upper GI Tract

An estimated 60 million Americans experience an episode of heartburn at least once a month. But for some 25 million Americans, heartburn is a daily occurrence. For about 10 percent of chronic heartburn sufferers, esophageal reflux eventually induces potentially dangerous cellular changes in the lining of the esophagus. In fact, according to at least one study, chronic heartburn causes an eightfold increase in the risk of developing esophageal cancer.

The painful, fiery sensations of heartburn are the result of stomach acids that have retrovulsed to invade the sensitive tissues of the esophagus. Normally, the lower esophageal sphincter (LES) muscle closes tightly to prevent this occurrence. When a faulty sphincter muscle is responsible for heartburn, the condition is referred to as gastroesophageal reflux (GERD). While antacids will help neutralize stomach acids and lead to temporary relief from heartburn pain, they do little to address the underlying cause or prevent future attacks. Moreover, chronic antacid consumption may dampen your defenses against harmful pathogens and even lead to dangerous mineral imbalances. Fortunately, there are a number of measures you can take to foster a more holistic and effective approach to the prevention and treatment of heartburn. A combination of natural remedies and lifestyle changes may even provide complete relief without the need for additional medication.

Obesity, caffeine, alcohol, cigarettes, and the consumption of acidic or fatty foods are all factors known to contribute to LES relaxation and GERD. Although many restaurants serve coffee at a piping 170°F to 180°F, drinking beverages exceeding 120°F to 130°F may actually damage your esophageal lining and weaken the lower sphincter. If you can't put your finger in a hot beverage without scalding yourself, it's too hot for your esophagus. Chewing gum after a meal may help neutralize stomach acids that have made their way into the esophagus. Avoid gum flavored with peppermint, however, as it triggers LES relaxation. And, because increased intra-abdominal pressure can also lead to reflux, limit the size of your meals and loosen your belt after eating.

Do you often feel drowsy after a meal? Rather than succumbing to post-prandial lethargy, take a leisurely stroll around the block. Light activity helps stimulate gut motility and digestion. If you are a heartburn sufferer, whatever you do, don't lie down for at least three hours after eating. And when you do finally hit the hay, harness gravity to help keep stomach acids from ascending into your esophagus while you sleep by elevating the head of your bed by six inches or by using a special foam wedge designed for heartburn sufferers. Sleeping on your left side may also provide relief.

To soothe irritated tissues and decrease esophageal inflammation, try drinking aloe vera juice two or three times daily. The B-complex vitamins choline, pantothenic acid, and thiamine can have long-term digestive benefits, including relief from chronic heartburn. Try them in combination (500 mg of choline three times a day, 1,000 mg of pantothenic acid twice a day, and 500 mg of thiamine once per day) for three to four weeks to see if your symptoms abate.

If symptoms persist, you may need a more complete diagnostic evaluation. See your doctor if you suffer from heartburn more than twice a week, experience difficulty swallowing, feel nauseated or vomit, or pass black stools.

The Lower GI Tract

Human intestines contain 100 trillion viable bacteria of several hundred different species. The resident bacterial flora of the large intestine comprise about 95 percent of the total cells in the human body (that's right—95 percent!), and they play a major role in health and nutrition. In the most basic terms, intestinal bacteria can be divided into two groups: species that are beneficial to host (human) welfare and species that are harmful to host (human) welfare.

Beneficial bacteria assist the body in a variety of physiological processes, including proper nutrient absorption and normal immune function. Certain forms of friendly bacteria may even help prevent food allergies, decrease your risk of developing colon cancer, and protect your intestinal lining against toxic injury. Harmful or pathogenic bacteria, on the other hand, produce toxic compounds that contribute to the development of malignant growths, liver and kidney disease, hypertension, atherosclerosis, reduced immunity, and premature aging. A growing number of scientists and health professionals believe that many "modern" diseases, including irritable bowel syndrome, Crohn's disease, ulcerative colitis, peptic ulcers, food allergies, and chronic fatigue syndrome, may be linked to colonization of the digestive tract by pathogenic bacterial strains.

Many factors can adversely effect the delicate balance of intestinal flora in favor of harmful microbes. And wouldn't you know it? These bad elements practically define Western living. Take us, for example. The American diet is rich in processed foods, chemical preservatives, and artificial ingredients. We drink chlorinated water, breathe polluted air, eat chemically treated produce, and consume unknown quantities of hormones and antibiotics in our meats. As a society, we extol the virtues of caffeine and have a penchant for nicotine and alcohol. We gulp down birth control pills, pain relievers, and countless other drugs like breath mints. We suffer from emotional stress, lack of exercise, and a low-fiber diet. These diet and lifestyle habits are catalysts that spell the demise of good bacteria. Is it any wonder we spend $15 billion every year on antacids and laxatives?

Now for the good news. The normal, healthy balance of intestinal flora may be restored through probiotics, or food supplements containing live microbes that beneficially effect the host animal by improving intestinal microbial balance. Probiotic organisms, which are found primarily in fortified milk and yogurt, include many "friendly" species of lactobacilli and bifidobacteria. Lactobacilli produce lactase, which hydrolyses lactose (milk sugar), increasing the digestibility of dairy products. Moreover, numerous animal studies have demonstrated that probiotic lactic-acid bacteria (LABs) such as lactobacillus and bifidobacteria can significantly increase the host's immune response to both infectious and carcinogenic challenges and may even confer protection against alcohol-induced liver disease and autoimmune disorders.

How can you be sure that you are consuming sufficient quantities of probiotics to achieve health benefits? The National Yogurt Association has established a "live active culture" seal to facilitate recognition by the consumer of yogurts containing adequate levels of viable cultures. In order to earn the seal, yogurt must contain 100 million active LAB per gram at the time of manufacture. Studies addressing the effects of probiotic bacteria on conditions like diarrhea, food allergies, and colon cancer typically find that an effective therapeutic dosage ranges between one and ten billion organisms two or three times per day. If yogurt isn't your thing, probiotic supplements are now available in the form of liquids, powders, capsules, and tablets. Choose brands that have research to back their products.

Another area of current research involves a newly defined class of compounds known as prebiotics, which represent an important adjunct to probiotics. Prebiotics selectively stimulate the growth and/or activity of health-promoting bacteria in the colon and help modify the gut flora in such a way that beneficial microbes (especially lactobacilli and bifidobacteria) become the predominant species. Prebiotics consist primarily of indigestible carbohydrates such as resistant starches, nonstarch polysaccharides (dietary fiber), unabsorbable sugars, and indigestible oligosaccharides. The most studied group of prebiotics are fructans, or fructose-containing oligosaccharides (FOS). Fructans occur naturally in onions, leeks, garlic, asparagus, bananas, artichokes, and other fruits and vegetables. In humans, administration of chicory fructans leads to the selective stimulation of the growth of the bifidobacteria. The colonizing cells of bifidobacteria produce short-chain fatty acids, which are bactericidal for certain pathogenic species. In addition, these short-chain fatty acids appear to promote the flow of blood through colonic vasculature, thereby improving colonic motility and increasing cell proliferation of the gut lining. The bottom line: improved nutrient absorption; decreased incidence of gas, bloating, and constipation; and a significantly reduced risk of developing colon malignancy.

Carbohydrates are not the only class of macronutrient that exerts prebiotic effects on the intestinal flora. In fact, researchers now believe that whey protein possesses prebiotic characteristics. This could explain why mice fed a whey protein diet mounted a far more vigorous immune response when exposed to carcinogens and lived five to six months longer than control subjects. In other studies, whey protein inhibited the growth of breast cancer cells in vitro. Even more encouraging, a regression in tumor size was observed when breast cancer patients ingested 30 grams of whey protein every day.

Though still in its infancy, the science of probiotics and prebiotics is assured a bright future in many industries. Experts hope that probiotic administration may eventually eliminate the need to add subtherapeutic doses of antibiotics to livestock feed. Even fish hatcheries have incorporated the use of probiotic supplementation with positive results. And because "friendly" bacteria acidify fermented foods to the extent that most harmful bacteria cannot grow, probiotics may one day represent an attractive alternative to chemical preservatives.

Unless you're a retired vegan teetotaler living on a remote mountain top, chances are good that your GI tract would benefit from a little rehab.

REVIEW Ten Steps to a Robust GI Tract

1. Avoid caffeine, alcohol, cigarettes, and the consumption of fatty foods.

2. If you can't put your finger in a hot beverage without scalding yourself, it's too hot for your esophagus.

3. To prevent excessive intra-abdominal pressure, eat frequent small meals and snacks (five or six a day) rather than the traditional two or three large ones.

4. Chew gum after meals to help neutralize stomach acid in the esophagus. (But avoid gum flavored with peppermint.)

5. Be sure your diet is high in soluble fiber. Apples, lentils, dried beans, peas, barley, citrus fruits, carrots, and oats contain significant amounts of soluble fiber.

6. Eat at least five servings of fresh fruit and vegetables every day. Emphasize fructan-containing foods like onions, leeks, garlic, asparagus, bananas, and artichokes.

7. Thoroughly wash all produce to avoid ingesting unnecessary contaminants.

8. Whenever possible, choose organically grown dairy products, meats, and produce.

9. Look for the National Yogurt Association's "live active culture" seal on yogurt products.

10. Select a quality whey protein to help meet your protein requirements.

MENTAL HEALTH MADE MANAGEABLE

Every year, an estimated 11 million Americans suffer from a major depressive episode, and that number is on the rise. Women are twice as likely as men to become depressed. It has been theorized that lower social status may, at least in part, provide an explanation for this epidemiological finding. The fact that women are more "in touch" with their feelings probably also contributes to the phenomenon. And monthly hormonal fluctuations certainly don't help!

The causes of depression are not completely understood. A familial tendency to experience depression indicates that hereditary factors may play an important role. In fact, in 50 percent of people who report recurrent episodes of depression, one or both parents also suffered depressive episodes. Typically, the first encounter with depression occurs in a person's twenties, thirties, or forties and may last for weeks, months, or even years. Individuals who are predisposed to mood disturbances usually experience several depressive episodes over a lifetime. Despite the fact that common catalysts include many organic (or physical) conditions, depression remains a fundamentally psychological manifestation. Arguably, the most compelling trigger for a depressive episode is the individual's unique life perspective, replete with the complex yet universal stresses she confronts on her day-to-day journey.

According to research, women, on average, feel less in control of their lives than men. Women are also more prone to ruminative coping mechanisms or, in other words, to dwelling on their negative sentiments. Ruminative coping is maladaptive because it adds to the stress that generated the negative feelings in the first place. The fact that women are more likely to embrace their negative thoughts than to take action to improve their situation often stems from perceived feelings of helplessness. The vulnerability provoked by inferior social status and its cohorts (which include low self-esteem and self-confidence) helps fuel feelings of helplessness, which in turn, add momentum to the vicious cycle of stress, depression, ruminative coping, helplessness, hopelessness, more stress, and even deeper depression.

The Overwhelming Role of Stress

In 1956, Viennese endocrinologist Hans Selye defined the three stages of the stress response to include an initial stage of alarm (the fight-or-flight response), an intermediate resistance stage, and the final stage of exhaustion. The initial alarm phase is controlled by the adrenal medulla and its hormonal mediators, most notably adrenaline. The alarm reaction typically involves an increase in heart rate and blood pressure in preparation for intense muscular activity. If stress is not conquered at this stage, the adrenal cortex takes charge of the situation. It secretes glucocorticoids (a class of steroid hormone) such as cortisol, which functions to regulate metabolic processes in response to continued stress. During the resistance stage, the supply of energy devoted to the brain and heart is increased by stimulating protein catabolism (muscle wasting) to liberate amino acids for gluconeogenesis (glucose production). In the absence of adequate coping mechanisms, the stress response progresses from resistance to exhaustion. The final exhaustion stage is fraught with illness, disease, and potentially death.

Despite this very clinical representation of the stress response, it does not take an enormous leap of faith to imagine the emotional sequelae of stress must, in many cases, contribute to subjective feelings of both anxiety and depression. The degree to which an individual experiences depression depends on numerous factors. Clinical depression, as defined by diagnostic medical criteria, includes the presence of at least four out of eight of the following symptoms:

- Changes in appetite with concomitant weight loss or weight gain

- Insomnia or hypersomnia

- Physical hyperactivity or inactivity

- Loss of interest in pleasurable activities

- Loss of energy and feelings of chronic fatigue

- Feelings of worthlessness or guilt

- Diminished ability to think or concentrate

- Recurrent thoughts of death or suicide

Left untreated, an episode of major clinical depression often lasts for six months or longer; dysthymia, a more mild form of depression, can last for years, even decades. Depressive episodes are usually managed with a combination of medication and psychotherapy. The three most commonly prescribed classes of drugs include tricyclic antidepressants, selective serotonin reuptake inhibitors (SSRIs), and monoamine oxidase inhibitors (MAOIs). A drug's effects usually take several weeks to be felt, and side effects are quite common. Tricyclics can cause sedation, weight gain, dry mouth, blurred vision, and sexual dysfunction. SSRIs often induce stomach upset, diarrhea, and headache. MAOIs can lead to dangerous elevations in blood pressure if taken with tyramine-containing foods or certain other medications. Psychotherapy can greatly enhance the effectiveness of medication. Even so, two-thirds of patients on long-term antidepressant drug therapy report dissatisfaction with their treatment.

There are numerous simple lifestyle choices that an individual can make to help alleviate or potentially prevent a depressive episode. Even if you have never suffered from depression or dysthymia, following these suggestions will probably have a significant and positive impact on your overall sense of well-being and also inspire improved stress management, increased energy levels, and reduced anxiety.

Rest and Recreation: Two Sides of the Same Coin

Many people restrict their allotment of sleep and exercise in order to squeeze more work into their busy schedules. While it may seem like a viable way to economize limited time, eventually this strategy backfires. Lack of sleep results in a sluggish disposition, as well as an increased incidence of depression, anxiety, and, of course, stress. Although it is certainly possible to survive on less, most people require a full eight hours of sleep for optimal health. Sleeping is not a sin! A good night's sleep will increase your productivity and more than make up for any time it takes from your work schedule.

Aside from all other health benefits, regular exercise clears the mind and invigorates the body, increasing productivity and general sense of well-being. According to a growing stockpile of research, regular exercise can help combat the negative effects of stress. Investigators used an animal model to show that exercise reduced both adrenal activity and brain levels of stress-related hormones.

Other lifestyle choices you should consider:

- Quit smoking. Studies have shown that smokers are more likely to suffer from depression, anxiety, and panic attacks.

- If your depression is seasonal, light therapy may help.

- Learn relaxation and stress-reduction techniques, such as yoga.

- Work on cultivating a positive attitude. Keep a journal, sketch, read, watch funny movies. Most important, treat yourself with kindness!

Diet: You(r Moods) Are What You Eat

It should come as no surprise that our eating habits have an enormous impact on how well we cope with stress. Dramatic drops in blood sugar cause the adrenal medulla to secrete adrenaline in order to liberate glucose stored in the liver. This adrenaline surge can mimic the symptoms of a panic attack and may actually induce an episode. You can avoid this scenario by making the effort to maintain stable blood sugar levels.

To prevent hypoglycemia, eat frequent, small meals throughout the day. Each meal should contain roughly the same proportions of protein and low-glycemic-index (LGI) carbohydrates. Whole grains, legumes, pasta, most fruit, and yams are all great sources of LGI carbohydrates. Sucrose, dextrose, alcohol, and exceedingly processed foods, such as white bread, contain high-glycemic-index (HGI) carbohydrates and are more likely to cause hypoglycemia. (See Chapter 2 for a more detailed explanation of the glycemic index and its relationship to hypoglycemia.)

Everyone, especially the nearly 10 percent of Americans who suffer from symptoms of chronic anxiety, should keep HGI foods to a bare minimum and would do well to avoid them altogether. If you find it impossible to eliminate these items from your diet, make an effort to always eat them in combination with LGI foods. This practice will serve to impede their absorption rate, functionally lowering their glycemic index. Other general dietary recommendations for good mental health include the following:

- Eat a high-fiber, low-fat diet rich in complex carbohydrates like fruits, vegetables, grains, legumes, soybeans, soy products, nuts, and seeds. Inadequate intake of complex carbohydrates may interfere with production of serotonin, a neurotransmitter closely associated with mood.

- For increased alertness, eat protein-rich foods with high essential fatty acid content such as salmon and white fish.

- Because gluten has been linked to depressive disorders, avoid wheat.

- Avoid alcohol, caffeine, refined sugar, and processed foods.

Supplementation

St. John's wort is a perennial plant that has been used for centuries in Europe to treat a wide variety of conditions, including depression, anxiety, insomnia, nerve pain, burns, and wounds. Though current studies indicate that its two main active ingredients, hypericum and pseudohypericum, may inhibit the AIDS virus, St. John's wort continues to gain recognition primarily as an alternative to standard antidepressant drugs. In Germany, it is the most commonly recommended first-line treatment for mild to moderate depression. In fact, recent German studies indicate that hypericum extracts from St. John's wort are just as effective as the widely prescribed antidepressant tricyclic drug imipramine for treating mild to moderate depression. And unlike imipramine, St. John's wort is virtually free of side effects. As a result, patients tolerate hypericum extracts much better than they do tricyclics, improving long-term compliance.

Like many prescription antidepressant medications, St. John's wort is believed to exert its influence through the seritonergic pathways (the channels in the brain that use the neurotransmitter serotonin) of the central nervous system. Several of its active ingredients have been demonstrated to inhibit monoamine oxidase, the enzyme responsible for metabolizing a number of neurotransmitters, including serotonin. By preventing serotonin breakdown, St. John's wort elevates central nervous system concentrations of this important mood-stimulating neurotransmitter. For the treatment of depressive symptoms, most sources recommend oral administration of 300 mg of St. John's wort extract (0.3% hypericum content) three times daily. It may take up to two months before the herb exerts a noticeable effect on mood, though many individuals report improvement after only two to three weeks.

Various sources also advise implementing the following daily supplement regimen for good mental health:

- B-complex vitamins: Take as recommended on the product label.

- Vitamin C: 500 to 1,000 mg two or three times a day.

- Vitamin E: 200 to 400 IU a day.

- Calcium: 1,500 mg a day.

- Magnesium: 1,000 mg a day.

- Zinc: 50 mg a day.

- Ginkgo biloba (24% ginkgo flavonglycosides): 80 mg a day.

- Chromium picolinate: 200 to 400 mcg a day.

- Essential fatty acids: 1 tablespoon of flaxseed oil (a good source of EFAs) a day.

CAUTION

If you are currently taking medication to treat depression, it is vital to consult your health care provider before altering your current drug regimen with either the addition of supplements such as St. John's wort or the discontinuation of your current therapy. Failure to consult your caregiver prior to exploring other treatment options can have serious, even deadly consequences.

REVIEW Ten Lifestyle Choices for Promoting Good Mental Health

1. Get enough sleep!

2. Exercise regularly.

3. Quit smoking.

4. Learn relaxation and stress-reduction techniques, such as yoga, and perform them daily.

5. Treat yourself with kindness!

6. Eat frequent, small meals.

7. Eat a high-fiber, low-fat diet rich in complex carbohydrates like fruits, vegetables, grains, legumes, soybeans, soy products, nuts, and seeds.

8. Eat protein-rich foods with high essential fatty acid content such as salmon and white fish.

9. Avoid alcohol, caffeine, refined sugar, and processed foods.

10. Implement a comprehensive supplementation regimen.

EATING TO COMBAT CANCER RISKS

According to the American Cancer Institute, one-third of all malignancies are directly related to diet. And wouldn't you know it? The same unhealthy foods that contribute to hyperlipidemia, cardiovascular disease, obesity, and hypertension also top the list as cancer-causing culprits. Just one more reason to avoid saturated fats, trans fats, and refined sugar. Fortunately, there are myriad delicious, healthy foods that have been proven to actually reduce cancer risks. For example, fruits and vegetables containing high concentrations of antioxidants like beta carotene and vitamins A, C, and E are especially effective at inhibiting tumor formation.

It all boils down to your food choices. Choose wisely and you may live longer!

Foods to Pursue

- **Blueberries.** Blueberries contain the highest concentrations of natural antioxidants of any food.

- **Broccoli sprouts.** Broccoli sprouts contain twenty times more sulforaphane than broccoli. Studies have linked the consumption of sulforaphane to the inhibition of tumor growth.

- **Citrus fruit.** The regular consumption of citrus fruit has been associated with a decreased risk of malignancy. This finding is probably associated with citrus's high concentration of the antioxidant beta-carotene. Ample dietary beta-carotene has been linked to a reduced incidence of numerous malignancies, including breast cancer, prostate cancer, lung cancer, melanoma, and bladder cancer.

- **Fish.** Fish contains high concentrations of omega-3 fatty acids, which are associated with a decreased risk for developing breast cancer.

- **Flaxseed.** Flaxseed contains isoflavones known as lignans that have been experimentally shown to inhibit the spread of malignant melanoma in animal studies. Lignans are believed to be beneficial in fighting cancer in general.

- **Garlic.** Garlic contains organosulfur, a phytochemical with beneficial antioxidant characteristics. According to one study, men who ate garlic at least twice a week were at decreased risk for developing prostate cancer when compared to men who abstained.

- **Green tea.** Green tea contains powerful polyphenolic antioxidants. The main polyphenol in green tea is epigallocatechin gallate (EGCG), which has been experimentally shown to inhibit tumor formation.

- **Pumpkin.** Cooked or canned pumpkin is one of the best natural sources of beta-carotene known to man.

- **Soy.** Mounting scientific evidence indicates that compounds contained in soy foods may reduce the risk of developing various cancers. Like flaxseed, soy is rich in lignan isoflavones and also in genistein, an isoflavone that has been shown to inhibit tumor growth in UV-exposed mice. Moderate soy consumption has also been demonstrated to have a protective effect against breast cancer.

- **Strawberries.** After blueberries, strawberries contain the second highest concentrations of natural antioxidants of any food.

- **Tomatoes.** Tomatoes contain very high concentrations of lycopene, a carotenoid in the same family as beta-carotene that has been shown to inhibit prostate cancer.

Soy as a Functional Food for Women

Soy protein is rich in phytoestrogens and isoflavones, which have numerous beneficial effects on human physiology and metabolism. Phytoestrogens are plant derivatives that structurally resemble human estrogen. Studies have demonstrated that the consumption of soy protein with its constituent phytoestrogens will delay menstruation by one to five days. This increase in cycle duration is largely due to an increase in the length of the follicular (egg development) phase. Since the mitotic rate (rate of cellular proliferation) for breast tissue is four times greater during the luteal (ovulation) phase, a lengthening of the follicular phase relative to the luteal phase is believed to confer protection against breast cancer, the second most common form of cancer in the West after colon cancer.

Breast cancer occurs five times more frequently in the United States than in Asia and Third World nations, where soy consumption is high. Indeed, Asian women have significantly longer menstrual cycles than Western women.

Phytoestrogens are also believed to decrease the severity of premenstrual symptoms and help regulate irregular menses. Moreover, they have been shown to reduce the incidence of menopausal symptoms such as hot flashes, as well as postmenopausal difficulties including heart disease, stroke, and osteoporosis. In one three-month study of post-menopausal women, those who consumed high concentrations of soy protein were shown to have increased bone density and stronger bones compared to those who received animal protein.

Research indicates that the beneficial influences of soy isoflavones effect both men and women and include a lesser risk of hypertension, a reduction in LDL (bad) cholesterol and triglyceride levels, and inhibition of the mutagenic cell processes that lead to various forms of cancer.

- **Walnuts.** Like fish, walnuts have high concentrations of omega-3 fatty acids.

- **Yogurt.** Yogurt contains live probiotic cultures that are believed to improve GI health and reduce the incidence of colon cancer.

Foods to Eschew

- **Butter.** It's high in saturated fat.

- **Fatty cuts of meat.** Fatty meats are high in both saturated fat and cholesterol.

- **Fried fare.** The oil these foods are fried in tends to be high in either saturated (animal) fat or hydrogenated trans fats.

- **Red meat.** Red meat is high in saturated fat and cholesterol. Even lean cuts of red meat slow gut motility.

- **Stick margarine.** Stick margarine is made with trans fats.

REVIEW Five Simple Steps to Sidestepping Cancer

1. Avoid a diet high in saturated fat, trans fats, and sugar.

2. *Do not* fry foods. Broil, bake, boil, microwave, steam, or roast them instead.

3. Remove visible fat from meat (and skin from poultry) before you cook it.

4. Eat at least five servings of fruits and vegetables every day.

5. Use naturally occurring nonhydrogenated oil (such as olive oil) for cooking.

PART II

Prescription for a Strong and Shapely Self

Muscle Up on Your Training IQ

The human body did not evolve to its present state of exalted beauty, superlative grace, and unequaled capability by adhering to a rock like a barnacle. Our ancestors did not lounge around in front of the campfire all day, rising only to fetch conveniently packaged, ready-to-eat chunks of woolly mammoth from the icebox. Like it or not, two or three generations of desk jobs can't eradicate millions of years of evolution. As a species, we thrive on physical exertion, and exercise is essential to both our physical and mental well-being.

In recent years, scientific investigation of human physiology and performance enhancement has subtly transformed the notion of "healthy." Fortunately, this metamorphosis has infiltrated cultural bias, including our subjective perceptions of beauty. In contemporary vernacular, "trim" no longer equates to "emaciated." "Attractive" is not synonymous with "lacking muscle." On the contrary! However, as anyone over the age of twenty will rapidly attest, a lean, toned, tantalizing physique does not just happen by magic.

WHY STRENGTH TRAINING BELONGS IN YOUR LIFE

A growing stockpile of scientific data has finally confirmed what any active person could have told you decades ago: The mental and physical benefits of regular activity are legion! And strength training is no exception. In addition to the obvious advantages of increased strength and a firmer, more shapely physique, weight lifting and other forms of resistance training have a wide spectrum of other immediate health benefits.

Strength Training Builds Muscle, and Muscle Burns Fat

It's as simple as that. Muscle is one of the most metabolically active tissues in the body. The more lean tissue (muscle mass) you possess, the more calories you burn, all day, every day, regardless of your activity level. In essence, your muscle actually helps eat your fat stores! How does this miracle occur? First, contracting your muscles requires substantial caloric expenditure. Every time you train, you burn calories. Second, exercise transiently raises your metabolic rate for several hours following each session. Hence, you continue to burn extra calories even if you're just lying on the couch watching TV. And finally, as alluded to earlier, studies have demonstrated that each pound of muscle that you possess requires approximately 35 calories per day just to exist. The more muscle you possess, the higher your resting metabolic rate, and the greater your overall caloric expenditure. Research indicates that for every 3 pounds of muscle gained by the average individual, resting metabolic rate increases by 7 percent, and daily caloric requirements increase by 15 percent.

Strength Training Helps Prevent Age-Related Metabolic Slowing

Adults who do not engage in regular resistance work will typically lose between five and seven pounds of lean mass every ten years. Although aerobic exercise improves our cardiovascular health and stamina, aerobic exercise alone cannot prevent age-related muscle loss. This fact alone has enormous bearing on why people tend to gain weight as they age. If, for example, a given individual were to lose 5 pounds of muscle over a decade, that would translate to roughly 175 (5 x 35 = 175) fewer calories that individual would expend each day. Assuming this individual's activity level and daily caloric intake were to remain constant over the ten years of gradual muscle atrophy, that would add up to a fat gain of more than 15 pounds during the tenth year alone!

Strength Training May Improve Cardiovascular Health

Although strength training does not substantially improve cardiovascular fitness (that's what aerobic activity is for), it does, nevertheless, seem to have a very positive impact on cardiovascular health. In several studies, regular strength training correlated to a reduction in both resting blood pressure and circulating triglyceride levels.

Strength Training May Improve Gastrointestinal Health

Just about every vigorous physical activity works to increase gut motility and, hence, decrease intestinal transit time (the time it takes for food to travel from your mouth to the toilet). Strength training is no exception. And according to several studies, the less time waste products linger in your bowel, the less likelihood you have of developing colon cancer.

Strength Training Decreases the Risk of Developing Osteoarthritis

Weight training increases the strength of not only muscles but also connective tissues, resulting in more resilient joints. Possessing stronger, more stable joints decreases your risk of injury, regardless of whether your typical day includes mountain climbing with a 40-pound pack strapped to your back or simply carrying a bag of groceries up your front steps. Strong muscles and joints are also essential to preventing the degenerative changes that can lead to osteoarthritis. But what if you already suffer from degenerative joint disease? According to several studies, moderate strength training (probably by virtue of its joint-stabilizing effects) actually helps ease arthritis pain.

Strength Training Decreases the Risk of Developing Osteoporosis

Undertaking resistance work and weight-bearing exercise is perhaps the single most effective way for a woman to prevent, and even reverse, the age-related decline in bone mineral density that can culminate in crippling osteoporosis.

Strength Training Improves Your Self-Esteem

Some scientists actually took the time (and money) to ascertain the existence of a phenomenon that seems blatantly obvious to me and anyone who's ever strolled through a gym during a busy afternoon: Strength training tends to improve a woman's self-esteem. Hello!

The scientists concluded that women gain self-esteem by mastering a physical challenge. While I'm sure that's part of it, I think the improved self-esteem has far more to do with feeling at ease with your body (and knowing you look good naked). Moreover, when you consider the collection of sordid characters you are bound to encounter during a lifetime (many of whom are men and at least some of whom will be bigger than you), it's empowering to realize that you possess the strength and confidence to put up a genuine fight, should the need ever arise. In fact, sociologists have demonstrated that a woman who moves with confidence is less likely to be singled out by a mugger or rapist as a prospective target.

REVIEW Seven Healthy Reasons to Hug Your Dumbbell

1. The more muscle you possess, the more calories you will burn, all day, every day, regardless of your activity level. In essence, muscle eats fat.

2. Without regular resistance training, the average person loses between 5 and 7 pounds of muscle every decade. This results in slowed metabolic rate and body fat accumulation.

3. Regular strength training correlates to a reduction in both resting blood pressure and circulating triglyceride levels.

4. Strength training may decrease your risk of developing colon cancer.

5. Strength training decreases your risk of developing osteoarthritis and has even been shown to reduce the pain of existing arthritis.

6. Strength training decreases your risk of developing osteoporosis and may even reverse osteoporotic bone changes.

7. Strength training boosts self-esteem and self-confidence.

DISPELLING MYTHS AND MISCONCEPTIONS

The degree to which taradiddles pollute the sphere of resistance training is nothing short of astounding. Women, in particular, have been deluged with stupid advice from unreliable, ill-informed, and sometimes downright malevolent sources (most of them male). During my years of involvement with the sports-fitness industry, legions of otherwise intelligent, educated women have approached me with shockingly misinformed concerns about weight training. Hopefully, the information contained within this book will serve as your personal weight-training panacea . . . a volume painstakingly composed to address your questions, allay your fears, and provide you with all the tools you will need to accomplish your every training goal. But, just for giggles, let's consider five of the most rampant and outrageous fables pertaining to women and weight training.

Myth #1: Strength Training Will Make Me Look Like a Man

The single largest obstacle between most women and their desire for a toned, healthy physique is masculophobia. Okay, I invented the word, but it doesn't change the reality of a completely ludicrous fear. Yes, strength training is essential for both women and men striving to optimize their muscular development. However, it's male hormones, not just the weight lifting, that enables the male of the species to build "manly" muscles, grow facial hair, and speak in low octaves.

Perhaps, like many of the misinformed, a night of insomnia lured you out of bed and into the living room for a relaxing session of channel surfing. While searching for something dull enough to induce sleep, you inadvertently found yourself wide awake, pulse racing, hands trembling, unable to tear your horrified gaze from the screen . . . no, it wasn't the Sci-Fi channel, it was just ESPN, rerunning footage shot at the Ms. Olympia Contest, the pinnacle of female bodybuilding.

Most women are appalled and dismayed by the Herculean she-creatures that inhabit the exotic world of women's bodybuilding. I understand why you might be put off from weight lifting after viewing such a spectacle. But you should know something about these women: With virtually no exception, every bodybuilder of any repute (male or female) self-administers enough anabolic hormones to dope a stable full of race horses. And even then, it takes years of dedicated training and enormous genetic potential for these "hormonally augmented" individuals to attain freakish muscularity, facial hair, and deepened voices. (More on women and steroid use in Chapter 8.)

The average woman possesses only a small fraction of the testosterone produced by the average man, which itself represents only a small fraction of the testosterone administered by the average professional bodybuilder. Exceptionally few women have either the genetic potential or sufficient amounts of natural testosterone to develop large muscles. Firm, toned, functional muscles? Absolutely! Bulging, large muscles? Dream on, ladies!

Even if you happen to be one of the genetically gifted, muscle takes work. It doesn't happen overnight. Should you ever feel that you are becoming too muscular, simple modifications to your training can temper your development. I will elaborate further on this issue in Chapter 7.

Myth #2: Strength Training Will Make Me Big and Bulky

This fear, commonly referred to (by me, anyway) as corpulophobia, is closely related to masculophobia. Many women avoid strength training because they fear weight gain and increasing limb girth. Many women are reluctant to train hard because, somewhere in the dark recesses of their misinformed subconsciousness, they believe they will wake up one morning, look in the mirror, and discover that they have transformed into a clumsy, cumbersome caricature of themselves.

As we learned in our discussion of myth #1, most women do not possess adequate testosterone to build muscles big enough to significantly increase their limb girth. In fact, for most women, the more muscle they build, the thinner their limbs become. How can that be? Simple: As your muscle mass increases, you expend a dramatically greater number of calories. In other words, your muscle literally burns the flab off your limbs. For the vast majority of women, the issue of bulk relates not to overly developed muscles but to overlying fat. Even a muscular individual will appear fat if she possesses enough adipose tissue to obscure the shape and definition of her lean tissue.

Say, for example, you were able to gain a pound of muscle for every pound of fat you lost. (This is pretty ambitious; I've found it generally takes three to four times as long to add a pound of muscle as it does to safely lose a pound of fat.) Although your total weight would not change, you would be thinner, because for every pound of fat you lose, you are actually losing three times the volume you would gain from an additional pound of muscle. In a nutshell, fat takes up a lot of space but doesn't actually weigh all that much. Muscle, on the other hand, takes up little space but is very heavy compared to fat.

I like to think of excess body fat as a jumbo-sized bucket of stale popcorn: tasteless, uncomely, bumpy, and voluminous. Then I imagine muscle as a living, growing, metallic framework, sinews of silver, gold, and platinum: strong, sleek, and exquisite in their complexity, yet functional and far weightier than popcorn. For the finishing touch, I visualize the precious metals devouring the popcorn to help fuel their growth.

Myth #3: Strength Training Will Make Me Slow and Torpid

Nothing could be further from the truth! Unless you train using an extremely low range of repetitions with very heavy weights, strength training will simply make you stronger, faster, more agile, and less prone to injury. (We'll examine the concept of appropriate repetition ranges in more detail later in this chapter.)

Myth #4: Effective Strength Training Takes an Enormous Time Commitment

Not so. The strength-training programs discussed in this book are guaranteed to provide you with visible, tangible results in just a few weeks. The required time investment for different routines ranges from about thirty minutes twice a week to a maximum of forty-five minutes three times a week.

Myth #5: If I Stop Weight Training, My Muscle Will Turn into Fat

Muscle tissue cannot transform into adipose (fat) tissue any more than your nose could transform into a third eyeball. Your muscles are highly differentiated organs, expressing very specific genetic properties, as reflected by their functional anatomy. Although fat is not nearly as complex as muscle in either form or function, it, too, is a differentiated end-stage tissue. Neither can become the other.

However, as is the case with many myths, if we closely examine this myth of muscle mutating to fat, we may discover in it a kernel of half-truth. You may recall that without the benefit of resistance training, the average adult can expect to lose at least 5 pounds of muscle per decade. You may also recall that every ounce of wasted muscle translates to an incremental decrease in metabolic rate, which typically is not compensated for by a proportional decrease in caloric intake. This dreadfully unfortunate, though entirely preventable, state of affairs leads to a substantial increase in body fat.

REVIEW Training Truths for Women

1. Strength training will not make you look like a man.

2. Strength training will not make you bulky.

3. Strength training will make you strong and agile, not slow and clumsy.

4. For rapid, visible, and tangible results, you need only two 30-minute sessions of strength training per week.

5. If you ever stop strength training, your muscles will shrink; they will not turn into fat.

BIOMECHANICS: A LESSON IN FORM AND FUNCTION

Biomechanics is the study of the material properties of biological materials. A basic understanding of musculoskeletal biomechanics and anatomy will help both decrease your risk of injury and maximize the effectiveness of your workouts. Fear not: You don't need an engineering degree (or even good grades in math) to master the following fundamental concepts.

There are three basic joint types: fibrous (like the sutures of the skull); cartilaginous (like the vertebrae and intervertebral discs); and synovial (as in the wrist, elbow, knees, and fingers). Synovial joints are surrounded by a fluid-filled space lined by a layer of tissue known as the synovial membrane. Muscles, tendons, ligaments, and cartilage surround, connect, and lend stability to the bones that comprise the joint. Injury to any of these structures may lead to pain, degenerative changes, and decreased range of motion. To prevent this from happening to any of your joints, let's begin by examining the concept of *viscoelasticity.* It's simpler than it sounds.

With virtually no exception, every tissue in the human body possesses viscoelastic material properties. In other words, when a deforming force is applied to a viscoelastic material, it will flow like a fluid (viscosity) and stretch like a spring (elasticity). Silly Putty is a perfect example of a viscoelastic material. Bones, ligaments, muscles, tendons, and cartilage all behave like Silly Putty when they are subjected to tensile forces.

Say you took a piece of Silly Putty and pulled it slowly. The Silly Putty would stretch or "flow" for some distance without breaking as long as you continued to apply a steady, tensile force. On the other hand, if you were to take this same piece of Silly Putty and yank on it, it would likely snap before stretching too far. The faster you try to stretch the Silly Putty, the stiffer it gets, the more force you must apply, and the easier it snaps. Hence, the rate of force application has a measurable effect on viscosity.

Now let's stick the Silly Putty in the refrigerator for a while. When we take it out and try to pull it, we have a hard time getting it to stretch. The colder the Silly Putty, the stiffer it becomes, the more it resists tensile forces, and the easier it snaps. Hence, temperature also has a measurable effect on viscosity.

Elasticity permits a material to recoil back to its original length after it's been stretched. For example, say you took a spring and stretched it to a new length. Within a certain range of stretching, the spring will return to its original length after the deforming force is removed. If you were to take this same spring and extend it beyond a certain limit, the spring sustains irreversible damage and no longer recoils fully once the force is removed.

The basic material properties outlined above have countless applications in the world of training and athletics.

REVIEW The Basics of Biomechanics

1. Virtually every tissue in the human body, including muscles, tendons, ligaments, and bones, possesses viscoelastic material properties.

2. When a deforming force is applied to a viscoelastic material, it will flow like a fluid (viscosity) and stretch like a spring (elasticity).

3. The faster you try to stretch viscoelastic material, the stiffer it gets, and the more likely it will sustain damage with the continued application of force.

4. The colder the viscoelastic material, the stiffer it becomes, and the more likely it will sustain damage with the continued application of force.

5. If you stretch a viscoelastic material beyond a certain limit, it sustains irreversible damage and no longer recoils to its original length once the deforming force is removed.

STRETCHING MAKES YOU STRONGER

Rule number one: Never tax a cold muscle. Remember what happened when the Silly Putty was refrigerated? Our muscles, tendons, and ligaments react in a similar manner. A "cold" muscle feels stiff and weak and, relative to a warm muscle, *is* stiff and weak. A warm tendon will accommodate more stretch without injury than a cold tendon will. And a cold ligament is far less likely to "flow" with the force. Before participating in any athletic activity, including stretching, drills, or weight training, you should raise your core (central) and peripheral (limb) body temperature. Get your heart beating and increase the blood flow to your extremities by participating in 5 minutes of a low-intensity cardiovascular activity. Try doing slow push-ups or take a brisk walk if you are on the field. Hop on the stationary bike or treadmill if you're at the gym.

Volumes have been written on the importance of stretching to promote strength and flexibility. Unfortunately, ignorance of basic musculoskeletal biomechanics precludes the modification of some archaic practices that involve dangerous stretching techniques. Despite overwhelming evidence supporting its benefits, far too many athletes fail to make stretching a significant part of their strength-training regimen.

By reducing muscle tension and promoting relaxation, stretching enhances the quality of recovery time, the period after exertion when muscle growth occurs. In theory, stretching loosens the fascial envelopes that form muscle compartments. This may lead to improved circulation and freer muscular development. In addition, consistent stretching helps prevent injuries by allowing for freer, more integrated movements. The increased body awareness that accompanies stretching makes it easier for the athlete to target a specific muscle or muscle group during an exercise. Believe it or not, regular stretching actually improves both strength and coordination. However, it is not enough to simply stretch. A basic knowledge of human physiology and tissue biomechanics can provide the athlete with all the tools necessary for proper stretching technique.

Stretching can be done with or without the aid of a partner. If you move your body into a stretched position, you are engaged in active stretching. In passive stretching, a partner provides the force to move into and hold the stretch. The two most basic stretching styles are referred to as static stretching and ballistic stretching. Static stretching involves moving slowly into a stretched position and holding that position for a desired period. This technique is simple to perform and safe for your joints. Ballistic stretching calls for sharp, rapid movements and utilizes the body's momentum to theoretically augment range of stretch. Ballistic stretching is unsafe and inefficient for two reasons. First, going back to our Silly Putty analogy, human tissue resists force when it is applied rapidly. Tendons and ligaments tighten when they are stretched too quickly. Tendons and ligaments will sustain injury at an earlier point if they are stretched rapidly than if they are stretched gradually. Second, a physiological phenomenon known as *protective reflex arc* causes your muscle to contract when your tendon senses a rapid length change. Your muscles will also contract in response to pain. It is obviously impossible to achieve a full stretch with contracted muscles! The take-home message is simple: Always stretch gradually to a point of mild discomfort, not outright pain. Never bounce. Instead, hold the stretched position for about 20 seconds.

Don't limit yourself to a pre-workout stretch. Continue to stretch frequently during your workout to promote circulation. It is especially important to stretch after your workout, when your muscles are hungry for glycogen replenishment. By increasing blood flow to a muscle, stretching will also remove waste products, such as lactic acid, from the muscles and help prevent soreness. In addition, more blood-borne nutrients are available for energy and growth.

There are countless different stretches designed to include the basic muscle groups. A detailed description of these techniques goes beyond the scope of this book. However, by following the general guidelines above, you can be assured that your stretching program will reap maximum benefits with little risk of injury.*

For more information on specific stretching techniques, I highly recommend
Stretching *by Bob Anderson (Bolinas, CA: Shelter Publications, 2000).*

REVIEW **Four Steps to Safe Stretching**

1. Before participating in any athletic activity, including stretching, drills, or weight-training, warm up with 5 minutes of a low-intensity cardiovascular activity.

2. Tendons and ligaments that are stretched rapidly will sustain injury at a point before the same tendons and ligament stretched gradually will.

3. Always stretch gradually to a point of mild discomfort, not outright pain. Never bounce. Instead, hold the stretched position for about 20 seconds.

4. Always stretch before, during, and after your workout.

WEIGHT-TRAINING BASICS

Weight training is an art that cannot be mastered overnight. I have seen world-class athletes walk into a gym and throw weights around with about as much finesse (and effectiveness) as a chimpanzee. For every correct way to perform an exercise, there are a dozen ways to do it wrong. Improper training techniques inevitably lead to injury, wasted hours, and an asymmetric physique. We all know people who spend their life in the gym and never seem to make any progress. These individuals could probably benefit from a couple of sessions with a competent personal trainer. Unfortunately, few of us can afford the luxury. Fortunately, it is entirely possible to teach yourself to train properly. Whether you are a world-class athlete or a phys-ed flunky, whether you've just invested in your first gym membership or have been training for years, the following basic weight-lifting tenets are guaranteed to maximize your gains and efficiency while minimizing your risk of burnout and injury.

Train Your Entire Body

A well-designed training program addresses all the major muscle groups. Full-body training prevents muscular imbalances that can lead to injury while also providing you with a proportioned, symmetrical appearance. All the sample routines included in this book fit the

What Is a Workout?

Most weight-training workouts include a combination of different exercises, each targeting a specific muscle or muscle group. The term "repetitions" (or "reps" for short) is used to describe the number of times you repeat a given movement without stopping to rest. The number of "sets" you complete is the total number of times you perform X number of repetitions. For example, say you did 15 tricep extensions followed by a 45-second rest, three times in a row. In weight-room vernacular, one would say that you had completed three "sets" of 15 "repetitions" of tricep extensions.

full-body bill. Once you attain the expertise and confidence necessary to orchestrate your own individualized program, always remember to place appropriate emphasis on all muscle groups.

Use Good Form

When you're learning to train with weights, you should make the movements of each exercise slowly and steadily, with strict attention to form. Concentrate on both the *concentric phase* (when the muscle is actively contracting) and the *eccentric phase* (when the muscle is relaxing back to its starting position) to maximize every repetition. Whether you are approaching full muscular contraction at the upper end of the motion range or full muscular relaxation at the lower end of the motion range, the weight's excursion through space should consist of an even, controlled deceleration to a full stop. Avoid sharp, jerky repetitions and using momentum to lift a heavy weight. These cheating tactics will not make you grow faster or become stronger, but they will place harmful stresses on your joint structures. Remember when we yanked on the Silly Putty? It acted as though it were stiff and brittle. Your muscles, tendons, and ligaments will do the same with the application of rapid force. Jerking the weight around will only lead to muscle shortening, decreased range of motion, and loss of flexibility.

I recommend using isometric tension to intensify the contraction at the peak of the excursion. This involves squeezing the contracted muscle for a half count before you begin the eccentric phase of the motion. This isometric squeeze, as it's called, will accentuate the muscular "pump," building additional strength and stamina. Likewise, be certain to relax completely and extend fully at the lower end of the excursion to avoid muscle shortening and weakness.

In general, it is helpful to exhale during the concentric phase and inhale during the eccentric phase. The two exceptions to this rule involve deltoid (shoulder) raises and most back exercises, for which the opposite breathing pattern should be implemented.

Learn to Isolate

Steady, controlled movements are the key to learning what it feels like to work a specific muscle or muscle group. After a few weeks of practice, even the novice can achieve the neuromuscular coordination necessary to identify and fully recruit muscle fibers from individual muscle groups. At this stage, you will be able to efficiently target these groups and minimize cheating with sympathetic muscles. Knowing the appropriate "feel" for working a particular muscle group will also enable you to use unfamiliar gym equipment or invent your own exercises for working that muscle group, simply by duplicating that feeling.

Start Your Workout with Power Movements

The initial set of the first exercise for each body part should be a light warm-up set. The warm-up set is intended not to tax the muscle but to promote circulation, raise the temperature of the involved tissues, and emphasize the mind-body connection so that you can better target specific muscles.

When the warm-up set is done, start your working sets. Begin with power movements, or multijoint exercises that target a large muscle group like chest, back, or glutes. Save for last the defining movements, or exercises that target a specific portion of a muscle group, such as the peak of the biceps. Defining movements should generally be performed at the end of your workout, after the bulk of your target muscle groups are already fatigued.

Use Appropriate Resistance within an Appropriate Repetition Range

The weight you lift must be heavy enough to challenge your muscles or you will make little progress. On the other hand, you should avoid extreme resistances, which put you at an increased risk for injury. How do you choose the correct weight for a particular exercise? If you're new to weight lifting, it's going to take a little trial and error. I recommend starting light and going for a high number of repetitions (20 to 30 per set). As I have already mentioned, it takes about three weeks for the novice to maximize the neuromuscular coordination necessary to identify and fully recruit muscle fibers from individual muscle groups. Once you've reached this stage, you should gradually increase the intensity of your training by progressing to heavier weights and a lower repetition range.

For effective progress, many sources recommend performing your working sets using approximately 75 percent of your single repetition maximum (SRM), or the greatest amount of resistance with which you can safely perform one repetition. Typically, 75 percent of your SRM corresponds to a repetition range of approximately 8 to 12. My personal recommendation is less restricted. For example, when you're targeting large muscle groups like chest and glutes with multi-joint power movements, it is safe and effective to use a repetition range as low as 6 or 7 per set (corresponding to about 80 percent of your SRM). Defining movements that target muscle fibers at the extremes of the motion range tend to be most effective when performed using a conservative repetition range of 12 to 15 per set (corresponding to about 70 percent of your SRM).

Depending on your specific aesthetic and athletic objectives, choosing the appropriate resistance and repetition range can become complicated—but not excessively so. We'll explore these variables in greater detail in Chapter 7.

Train Your Muscles to Fatigue

The objective of resistance training is not to take a preconceived amount of weight and complete a preconceived number of repetitions. I see a lot of people who have adopted this particular method. I call them "gym zombies." These misguided souls drift like blank-faced automatons from one exercise to the next, never straying from their established route. At each station, they choose the identical weight as the week before, complete exactly 10 repetitions (never more, never less), and resume their tedious course. These rueful plebes often train for months (or even years), never fully grasping why their strength never increases, why their physique never improves, and why they find going to the gym such a dull, monotonous affair.

Whether you are a power or endurance athlete, an ectomorph or mesomorph, a novice gym-goer or an elite athlete, your fundamental weight-training goal is the same: to induce muscular hypertrophy (growth) and strength gains by fatiguing your muscles. *Muscle fatigue* occurs during an exercise set once you have completed the greatest number of repetitions possible, using good form. If you don't train to the point of muscle fatigue, your progress will be short-lived, and you will soon find yourself stumbling down the dreaded path of the gym zombie.

Make Gradual Progress for Safe Gains

Every strength-training program needs a protocol for safe, effective progress. Eventually, most people develop an intuitive sense of how and when they should increase their training intensity. Until that happens, I recommend adding about 5 percent resistance whenever you are able to perform a given movement, with good form, for at least one repetition in excess of your target range for that exercise.

Mix It Up

Even the most brilliantly designed training program will gradually lose its efficiency. In simple terms, your body is too smart for its own good. As you become more and more adept at performing a particular movement, the results you get from that movement will reach a plateau. It's time to mix things up. Your entire work out should be modified every few weeks for best results. I urge you to constantly try new exercises to add to your repertoire. Look around the gym. Talk to people. Consult magazines. Experiment on your own: Change bench angles, alter foot stances, switch the order of your exercises, try super sets or strip sets, and so on. Be creative. We'll discuss this topic in greater detail in Chapter 7.

Listen to Your Body

Overtraining is the second most common mistake (bad form being the first) I see in the gym. Human beings come in an enormous vari-

Muscle Fatigue versus Muscle Failure

The concept of *muscle failure* is similar to that of *muscle fatigue*, with one subtle, albeit important, difference. Muscle failure occurs during an exercise set *after* you have completed the greatest number of repetitions possible, using good form. In order to reach muscle failure, either you need a partner to assist you or you must "cheat" with momentum and/or improper form in order to squeeze out the last couple of repetitions. I never recommend that beginners work their muscles to failure. This technique has the potential to result in enormous microtrauma and delayed-onset muscle soreness. Moreover, if you don't know how to "cheat" properly, you risk injury. Working muscles to failure is most appropriate for those who wish to make maximal size, strength, and power gains and have little regard for local endurance. This type of training is most appropriate for power athletes and hard-gaining ectomorphs.

ety of shapes, colors, and sizes. Human physiology, however, is fairly uniform. As a rule, natural athletes (by natural, I mean those who do not abuse anabolic steroids) do not benefit from directly training the same body part with high intensity more than once a week. If you find yourself losing enthusiasm for your workouts, if you are constantly tired, or if your progress has slowed or stopped, it's time for a break. If you have been training consistently, I recommend taking a week off every two to three months. You will return to the gym reinvigorated, renewed, and rested. You will not lose strength in one week. Even after a month off, chances are you will surprise yourself by returning to the gym stronger than when you left. (See also Chapter 8.)

Be Patient

Rome wasn't built in a day, and you won't be either. You will, however, see progress if you are patient and stick with it! No two physiques are exactly the same, so you cannot measure your progress against that of others. Many people are frustrated by the difficulty they encounter losing those last few pounds of fat. Lean people are discouraged by how long it takes them to put on weight. Physique athletes are constantly balancing the tasks of building muscle mass and achieving maximal definition. You can have both if you stick to the basic principles outlined above, train consistently, and give yourself time. Why don't you take some photos now and compare them to how you look three months from now? I guarantee you will be amazed by the progress you've made.

REVIEW Thirteen Tips to Top Technique

1. Train your entire body.

2. Always employ proper form. Concentrate on both the concentric and eccentric phases to maximize every repetition.

3. With the exception of deltoid raises and back exercises, exhale on the concentric phase of the movement and inhale on the eccentric phase.

4. Learn to isolate specific muscles.

5. Warm up with an initial light set of each exercise.

6. Begin training sessions with multijoint power movements. Finish with higher repetitions of defining movements.

7. Choose the appropriate repetition range to accommodate the particular exercise. If you're new to resistance training, start with light weights and a high repetition range.

8. Train muscles to fatigue.

9. Train each muscle group once per week.

10. Implement a gradual progression in training intensity for safe, steady gains.

11. Maximize your body's response by giving it new challenges.

12. Avoid overtraining.

13. Be patient!

THE LATE, GREAT, WEIGHT BELT DEBATE

For a preponderance of training authorities, the venerable weight belt holds a most revered status. Recently, however, the sports science community has raised doubts as to the efficacy and even the safety of training with weight belts.

To better understand how a weight belt provides low back support while improving performance, we must examine the body's natural mechanisms for spine stabilization. The largely fluid contents of the abdominal cavity are surrounded and held in place by a girdle of muscle. The intra-abdominal pressure (IAP) created by this muscular arrangement results in a mechanical force, described as hoop tension, that buttresses and stabilizes the spinal column. A tightly cinched weight belt enhances the effects of hoop tension, thereby reducing the compressive forces on the lumbar discs by as much as 50 percent. Studies have further demonstrated that a weight belt contributes to faster lifting movement, greater hip extension relative to knee extension (hence reducing knee strain), and increased subjective comfort. It sounds too good to be true! And it is . . .

When you lift with the assistance of a weight belt, your trunk muscles don't work as hard. Reliance on the belt eventually deconditions the stabilizing musculature, with concomitant muscular atrophy.

Moreover, weight belts restrict the range of motion in the lumbar spine. Both flexion/extension (bending) and rotation (twisting) are affected. When you flex your lower back to lean forward, 80 percent of the motion normally occurs between the fourth and fifth vertebrae (L4 and L5) of the lumbar spine. The substantial, repetitive forces endured at L4–L5 explain why it is the most commonly injured segment of the low back. The presence of a weight belt restricts motion at higher lumbar levels, forcing virtually all movement to originate at L4–L5 and placing enormous additional strain on this already vulnerable region. The combination of deconditioned trunk muscles and increased lumbar stress leads to excessive wear and tear—a sure way to accelerate disc degeneration and cause injuries.

Heavy reliance on a weight belt has other far-reaching consequences. It impedes diaphragmatic breathing, and the resulting "chest breathing" is associated with tension headaches, poor posture, degenerative changes in the cervical discs, and, eventually, the development of a barrel chest. Use of a weight belt may also impede blood flow to the heart and raise blood pressure.

No matter how you look at it, the disadvantages of "buckling up" outweigh the benefits. Weight-lifting competition, for which the belt's purpose is instantaneous performance enhancement, and not muscle building, most warrants the use of a weight belt. If you insist on wearing one at the gym, do not wear it at all times. Don the belt solely for those exercises that require the spinal erectors (the muscles that support the spine) to work against high resistance, such as the squat and dead lift. Refrain from relying on the belt for intensities below 80 percent of your SRM. Loosen the belt between every set to ensure restoration of normal breathing patterns.

Unraveling the Mystery of Knee Wraps

Like their nefarious cousin the weight belt, knee wraps work through the compressive mechanical force known as hoop tension. The tightly applied wrap creates an extension force in the knee joint while pinning the quadriceps tendon to the femur for better leverage. This process can impart a 5 to 10 percent increase in SRM during squats. In addition, wrapping a knee stabilizes the joint and reduces the shear forces generated by the quads on their tendinous attachments to the patella (knee cap) and tibia (shin bone). This process decreases the risk of avulsion injuries, in which the muscle literally tears away from the bone.

Unfortunately, knee wraps confer support by removing stress, thereby limiting the adaptive response of the joint structures. Simply stated, wrapping the knees prior to an exercise reduces overall stimulation of the involved muscles, tendons, and ligaments. Hence, if your primary goal is injury-free muscular development, as opposed to record-breaking poundages, you might consider keeping the wraps under wrap altogether.

In general, like the weight belt, knee wraps are most appropriate when used for instantaneous performance enhancement. Their limited application includes powerlifting meets and squatting in a range that exceeds 80 percent of your SRM. As Dr. Fred Hatfield of the International Sports Science Association points out, wearing wraps while squatting below this intensity is "counterproductive to providing the adaptive overload" necessary to stimulate a beneficial response in the tissues comprising the knee.

Solving the Riddle of Wrist Straps

The object of wrist straps is not to eliminate the gripping effort but, rather, to assist the forearm flexors in the performance of a movement for which grip strength is a limiting factor. Without grip assistance, the set must be terminated prematurely, cheating target muscle groups out of growth-stimulating repetitions.

I advise the beginner to refrain from using straps altogether in order to maximally stimulate the untrained forearms. The more experienced lifter should apply wrist straps only at high intensities, and as necessary. Some lucky individuals are genetically predisposed to amazing forearm strength and never need to use this piece of training gear. For the rest of us, the judicious use of wrist straps can be a great addition to the lifting arsenal.

I also recommend including a few sets of forearm-specific exercises in your standard training regimen to ensure optimal forearm development, even with the occasional use of wrist straps.

To correctly apply wrist straps, position the loop in the palm of your hand with the thick, stitched side facing up. Close your fingers around it. With your other hand, wrap the running end of the strap across the thenar eminence (heel of your thumb), around the back of your wrist, and across the hypothenar eminence (heel of your hand). Then thread the end through the loop so that the remainder of the strap extends from between the thumb and index finger. Repeat these steps with the opposite hand. Now, with your palms facing down, coil the running ends of the straps securely around the thumb sides of the bars.

Slap On Those Gloves!

Athletic gloves come in myriad shapes, colors, and materials, including leather, sheepskin, cotton, spandex, and neoprene. Unlike the other types of training gear we've discussed, athletic gloves have few disadvantages. In short, gloves increase relative grip strength by decreasing hand discomfort and absorbing sweat. They also help prevent callous formation by reducing friction. If you choose to wear rings while you train, gloves will protect your fingers as well as your rings.

Newer glove designs may include built-in wrist straps, neoprene pads with and without finger separation, and adjustable pads that attach to supportive wristbands. Find a pair that suits your preferences; your hands (as well as your significant other) will thank you.

REVIEW Training Aids

1. Skip the weight belt unless you are a competitive power lifter.

2. Skip the knee wraps unless you are a competitive power lifter.

3. The judicious use of wrist straps can be a great addition to the lifting arsenal. However, the beginner is advised to refrain from using straps in order to maximally stimulate the untrained forearms.

4. Gloves increase relative grip strength by decreasing hand discomfort and absorbing sweat. They also help prevent callous formation by reducing friction. Wear them!

Designing Your Routine

For those who view the gym as a place only slightly less mysterious than outer space, take heart: By the time you're done with this book, even if you retain only 10 percent of everything you've read, you will know more about strength training than the average dedicated gym-goer. And you will have the remaining 90 percent at your fingertips. I encourage you to refer to this book often during your journey, both to refresh your memory and to deepen your understanding of complex topics.

However, even if you were to master intellectually all the concepts contained in the following pages, without practical application, your understanding of strength training would remain very limited and one-dimensional. The longer you train, the more palpable these chapters will become. I won't lie to you: Training will feel awkward at first. But what begins as a simple, perhaps even clumsy physical expression of mental data eventually will manifest as a tangible, corporal reality.

To the uninitiated, the remarkably acute mind-body connection engendered by athletic training can seem almost supernatural. Think of the extraordinary feats of physical prowess demonstrated by gymnasts, dancers, and martial artists, who use nothing more than their bodies to defy gravity. As with any athletic activity, your knowledge of strength training will eventually transcend your conscious intellect to become part of your subconscious awareness. You will simply "know" what to do without even thinking. The process may take months or even years. But the rewards are priceless. Long before you fully master strength training, you will delight in the pleasures of feeling the clock turn back. You will revel in soaring energy levels, feel the power of your expanding strength, and discover a well of untapped vitality deep within yourself. One day you will awaken to discover that you have regained the healthy vigor of times long past, and an enviable physique to boot!

USING THIS BOOK TO DESIGN A ROUTINE

This chapter explains several different types of strength-training routines, as well as the rationale behind why you might choose one over another. When you're ready to begin strength training, you'll be asked to turn to Appendix C to choose the routine that best fits your schedule, your workout history, and your current fitness level. The routine you select from Appendix C lists the recommended number of sets and repetitions for resistance exercises—power movements and, if applicable, defining movements—you will use to train specific muscle groups. As you'll learn in Chapters 9 through 12, each muscle or muscle group responds to a variety of muscle-specific exercises. Dozens of these muscle-specific exercises are listed by category in Appendix D. With your Appendix C routine in hand, you'll turn to Appendix D and select the particular muscle-specific exercises you will perform to satisfy the demands of your chosen routine.

KEEPING A JOURNAL

I recommend that everyone use a training journal to facilitate workouts. This is especially important if you are new to the weight room. It will take a few weeks before you get your bearings. Record the resistance you used and the number of repetitions you were able to complete for each set. This saves time and guesswork during your next session.

By accurately charting your progress, you will know at what point to "go heavier." You will also have written documentation should you hit a training plateau or start to backslide. A training plateau may signal that your routine has lost effectiveness and is in need of an overhaul, whereas regression is often an indication of overtraining.

HOME TRAINING

Ironically, many women are so self-conscious about being out of shape or overweight that it actually prevents them from joining a gym. Many others, especially those who have never before embraced the joy of physical activity, feel horribly intimidated by the gym atmosphere, like cold-water fish flopping about on a hot sidewalk. This is completely understandable. However, I urge you not to permit an irrational fear of the gym to derail your very bright future!

If you would prefer not to begin your very personal journey in front of a bunch of strangers or in alien surroundings, rest assured, you can make great progress at home with a minimal investment of space and money. Essential equipment includes the following:

- A pair of 5-, 8-, 10-, 12-, 15-, and 20-pound dumbbells

- A single, adjustable barbell or a set of barbells ranging from 20 to 50 pounds

- An adjustable bench (both decline and incline is optimal, though incline alone will suffice)

- A chin-up bar mounted in a door frame

Of the movements explained in Chapters 9 through 12, numerous examples require nothing more than the above-mentioned gear. These "home-friendly" exercises are clearly indicated as such.

REVIEW **Essential Equipment for Every Home Gym**

1. Multiple sets of dumbbells

2. An adjustable barbell

3. An adjustable bench

4. A chin-up bar

TRAINING AT THE GYM

There's an awful lot to be said for belonging to a health club or gym. It gets you out of the house and away from the office, to a "neutral" space where you can temporarily escape the distractions of family and career to concentrate on your workout. After you've belonged to the same gym for a few weeks, it's difficult not to experience a sense of fellowship with the other members. I don't mean these individuals will necessarily become part of your social circle. Beyond weight lifting, spin class, or kickboxing, you may not have a shred in common with any single member of this eclectic gathering. Nevertheless, for several hours of every week you become part of an assembly of individuals brought together under one roof by a powerful compulsion: the pressing need for physical challenge.

This commitment to exertion ignites a sort of tacit camaraderie, a phenomenon I term "collective dedication." If you can tap into this force, you may discover a remarkable source of motivational energy. Even wearing headphones and training solo, I always feel inspired to be in the proximity of other sweaty, like-minded individuals. In addition, a health club or gym is the ideal place to meet prospective training partners, learn new techniques, increase your exercise repertoire, and join classes. Plus, training at a gym is far more entertaining than training alone.

Selecting a gym is a serious undertaking that you should approach like any other major life decision. Choose your gym like you would your spouse! In determining your gym compatibility, consider the three Cs: cost, convenience, and climate.

Cost

Can you afford to join the gym of your choice? Frankly, in my opinion you can't afford not to. It's worth a few extra dollars if the expenditure ensures that you will train faithfully. I know far too many individuals who were lured blindly into a bad gym relationship by limited time offers. If you feel lukewarm toward a club, I guarantee that your motivation to train consistently will be lukewarm as well.

Convenience

Convenience should be a top priority. In today's high-pressure world, almost everyone is struggling to negotiate a hectic schedule. The gym of your choice should be no more than a few miles from your home or work. In the evening after a long day at the office or in the morning after a too-short night's sleep, it is a thousand times more difficult to feel inspired about a workout if the trek to the gym exceeds 15 minutes.

One other consideration: How does your schedule jibe with the gym's? Are there times of the day that the gym is too crowded to permit a decent workout? If you have an unusual routine, is the gym open during odd hours? Don't make the mistake of evaluating your prospective club on a lazy Sunday morning if you intend to train between 6:00 and 8:00 P.M. on weekdays.

Climate

Numerous intangibles contribute to the atmosphere of a gym, which is as important as any other factor in determining your gym compatibility. When it comes to choosing a gym, I strongly recommend living in sin before you march down the aisle. If the club you're considering does not offer a short-term (say, two-week) membership, I would regard it with some suspicion. A health club worth its salt does not rely on high-pressure salespeople who descend like vultures on every walk-in, hungry to close the deal. A good club depends more on positive referrals than on membership drives, and most gyms will not object to potential members "testing the waters" before committing to a long-term membership.

To evaluate whether a gym's climate is appropriate for you, examine your priorities. Are you looking for a health club primarily for weight reduction or cardiovascular health? Then pay special attention to the aerobic facilities. Let's face it, nobody likes cardio workouts. The best way to stay committed to fat burning is to make it as interesting as possible. Does the gym offer aerobics, spinning, dance, slide, or other classes guaranteed to lesson the cardio burden? Does the stationary equipment have beverage holders, stands for reading material, or, better yet, a cardio theater with headphone outlets? Is there a variety of cardio equipment? Can you abandon the LifeCycle when your butt becomes sore and try the treadmill or the stairclimber instead? Is the equipment ample enough to accommodate members during peak hours? Is it generally in good repair and working order?

If you are serious about building muscle, choose a gym with excellent weight machines and a complete set of both dumbbells and barbells. Check that the cable stations pull smoothly and have a variety of attachments. The presence of Cybex, Icarian, Flex, and/or Hammer equipment is a good sign. If you find nothing but old Nautilus machines or hydraulic contraptions, this is a bad sign. If certain "bonus" services are of special importance to you, try not to settle for less. If you like to swim after a weight workout, join a gym with a pool. If you have kids in tow, find a gym with child-care facilities. If you want to bring your own personal trainer, be sure the gym will allow this practice. If you must have a protein drink the minute you finish a workout, join a gym with a juice bar.

REVIEW Vital Tips for a Good Gym Union

1. When comparing costs, remember it is worth a few extra dollars if the expenditure ensures that you will train faithfully.

2. The gym of your choice should be no more than a few miles from your home or work.

3. Give your prospective gym a test drive before joining.

4. Examine your training priorities and be certain that your gym can provide you with everything necessary to meet your objectives.

FOR THE BEGINNER

The most crucial first step in starting your training program is being honest with yourself when answering the following question: How much time do I realistically have to exercise? Radical lifestyle changes are difficult to commit to, but a gradual evolution is unlikely to send your system into shock. Underestimate rather than overestimate the time you are willing to spend in the gym or training at home. As the weeks go by, it's simple to add to your routine. However, if you start your new program by missing scheduled workouts, you are liable to become discouraged and give up.

Baby Steps

According to the National Health and Nutrition Examination Survey, 24 percent of American adults are completely sedentary and 54 percent don't spend adequate time exercising. In addition to burning calories while you exercise, regular physical activity increases your metabolic rate so that you burn more calories even while at rest. Regular exercise also lowers your heart rate, blood pressure, and cholesterol levels while increasing your energy levels.

Even if you have never been physically active in your life, it's never too late to get healthy. Walking, combined with a basic full-body strength-training routine, is a great way to begin. Although walking does not impose the same high-impact stresses as running, it is still very important to invest in quality footwear that offers proper ankle support and a well-cushioned sole. Under your doctor's supervision, start with a reasonable goal, such as 10 to 15 minutes of brisk walking five or six days a week. As your fitness level improves, work your way up to 30 to 40 minutes five or six days a week. When this is no longer challenging, graduate to walking hills, stairs, or sand for added resistance. Eventually, you may want to advance to running, biking, roller blading, cross-country skiing, team sports, and beyond. (We will return to the importance of cardiovascular training in Chapter 8.)

And Now for Strength Training!

Spending as little as 25 minutes twice a week working with weights will give you visible, tangible results. If you are currently leading a fairly sedentary existence, be aware that the ligamentous laxity and muscle shrinkage, or atrophy, that result from inactivity will render your joints vulnerable to injury. Even if you are currently active in other sports, taking up weight lifting will involve using muscles and joints in untested and different ways. To help avoid injury and mitigate as much early muscle soreness as possible, it is of utmost importance that you begin your training gradually.

As you may recall from Chapter 6, directly training any muscle group (with the notable exception of the abdominal muscles) with high intensity more than once a week is overtraining. If you have never trained with weights or have taken a significant break from weights, I do not recommend training at maximum intensity right away. Training to the point of complete muscle exhaustion or muscle failure (versus muscle fatigue; see page 99) during the first crucial workouts will result in tremendous muscle soreness, and you may never return. I advise you to start slowly by implementing a full-body routine consisting of two or three sets of movements for every major muscle group. I also recommend using relatively light weights and a high repetition range (15 to 20 reps).

REVIEW Practical Suggestions for the Beginner

1. Work up to a minimum of five cardiovascular training sessions of 30 minutes duration per week.

2. Underestimate rather than overestimate the time you are willing to spend weight training.

3. If you have never trained with weights or have taken a significant break from weights, start with light weights for a full-body workout, and increase your intensity slowly.

THE FULL-BODY ROUTINE: PROGRESS AT YOUR OWN PACE

The full-body routine combines several attributes that are especially salient for the beginner. First, it calls for a minimum time commitment, which can be extremely beneficial while you adapt to the scheduling demands of regular exercise. Second, full-body routines are less physically taxing than the more advanced split routines. Let's face it: It's practically impossible to learn something if you're exhausted. The reduced intensity of a full-body routine will leave you with enough energy during your workout to master the basics. And third, if you are a novice weight lifter, a full-body routine should minimize excessive muscle soreness and provide your body with ample opportunity to recover between your initial workouts.

Although I feel it is very important to embark on your strength-training career using the most basic full-body routine, you should allow yourself the freedom to progress at your own pace. For example, say you begin your training using Full-Body Routine A described in Appendix C, which requires 25 to 30 minutes twice a week. After a week or two, you may wish to increase the intensity of your program by adding a third weekly session. Or you may wish to move on to Full-Body Routine B, which increases the intensity of your training with additional sets for each muscle group and requires about 45 minutes twice a week. Of course, if you are satisfied with the progress you are making with two weekly sessions of Full-Body Routine A, you should feel free to stick with it indefinitely.

Now let's try a dry run. Let's say you turn to Appendix C to choose a full-body routine and decide that you want to start with the minimum time commitment espoused by Full-Body Routine A: two weekly training sessions of 25 to 30 minutes' duration. The description of Full-Body Routine A lists the major muscle groups you will train and the types of movements you will use to train them. Before trekking to the gym or dragging out your exercise equipment, you would choose the specific movements you intended to use from Appendix D and record them in a notebook or training journal. Then you would train each muscle group by performing 15 to 20 repetitions of the chosen exercise (that makes one set), resting, and repeating the exercise (that makes two sets). After completing a total of two sets per major muscle group, you would have survived your first training session.

REVIEW Working through a Full-Body Routine

1. Full-body routines take less time, are less physically taxing, and result in less muscle soreness than split routines.

2. Choose the exercises you intend to do before starting the workout.

3. Progress at your own pace.

4. Chart your early progress with a training journal. Record your exercise choices as well as the amount of weight you used and the number of repetitions you were able to complete with good form.

SPLIT ROUTINES FOR MORE MUSCLE

Unlike a full-body routine, which works all the major muscle groups in a single session, a split routine targets only a portion of the body in a single session, usually addressing the entire body over two or three weekly workouts. A split routine does not necessarily require lengthier sessions than a full-body workout. It does, however, demand a significantly greater training intensity.

The recommended repetition range for a full-body workout is relatively high, on the order of 15 to 20. A high repetition range necessitates using a relatively light resistance, on the order of 50 to 70 percent of your single repetition maximum (SRM). This high-rep/light-resistance approach decreases your risk of injury while you build confidence, strength, and coordination in the weight room. Even the least intensive full-body routine will produce a firmer, more toned appearance and measurable strength gains in just two to three weeks. However, high-rep/light-resistance training becomes less efficient as your strength and conditioning improve. If you arrive at a point where you want to accelerate your progress and build lean tissue more rapidly, you will need to use heavier weights combined with a lower repetition range.

For example, by training at 70 to 80 percent of your SRM, you can expect muscular fatigue to occur within 6 to 15 repetitions. However, it's just about impossible to train your entire body with that degree of intensity without passing out or losing your lunch. Your body simply isn't enough blood and glycogen to go around. Here's where the split routine comes into play. After all, why would you want to cram all your training into a single, agonizing, three-hour session guaranteed to leave you feeling queasy and sore for days

What's So Special about the Zones?

Once you have perused the various split routines listed in Appendix D, you may wonder about the rationale behind dividing the body into these particular zones. Rest assured, there is a method to my madness. Even with perfect form and focus, it is physiologically impossible to fully isolate a solitary muscle to the exclusion of all others. When you are performing an exercise that targets a particular muscle or muscle group, there will always be some degree of recruitment from synergistic and agonistic muscle groups (groups of muscles that work together as a unit or in tandem to accomplish single- or multijoint movements). During a session of intense high-resistance/low-repetition training, target muscle groups sustain significant microtrauma and typically require a full week to recover. Hence, by grouping synergistic muscles together in the same session, each split routine is structured to avoid training overlap.

For example, following a session of high-intensity arm training on Monday, ideally, your biceps and triceps should be kept out of commission for a full week. But say you then wanted to train your chest muscles on Wednesday. Unfortunately, many of the exercises used to target your pectoral muscles also call for significant triceps input. Hence, you would inadvertently retrain your triceps before they've had adequate time to fully recover, and this will serve only to delay muscle healing and inhibit your progress. Why train for detrimental results? Instead, you should have trained your chest muscles at the same time that you trained your triceps; this would allow these synergistic muscles to rest at the same time. The zones of the split routines in Appendix D are carefully mapped to accommodate synergistic and agonistic muscles.

when, instead, you could "split" your body into smaller zones and devote a 30- to 60-minute session each week to each zone?

By narrowing your focus to a handful of muscle groups per training session, you can dramatically accelerate your progress without dramatically increasing the time you need to train. If you decide to graduate to a split system, start with the split routine that requires roughly the same time commitment as your current full-body routine. For example, Full-Body Routine A just happens to correspond to Split Routine A, with two 25- to 30-minute sessions per week. Likewise, Full-Body Routine B corresponds to Split Routines B. Split Routine C takes it up a notch. Split Routines D and E, which call for three weekly sessions of 45 to 60 minutes, may prove too arduous for the beginner. They reflect the maximum volume of weight training I advise for a natural athlete. (By natural, I mean steroid-free.) Higher volumes of resistance work can overcome the body's ability to recover completely between sessions. This leads to fatigue, chronic muscle soreness, stunted progress, and an increased risk of injury. In a word, overtraining. I advise adopting either Split Routine B or Split Routine C for at least two to three weeks before progressing to D or E.

The Two-Day Split

The two-day upper/lower body split is fairly self-explanatory. In my opinion, it is also the most effective two-day split routine. Although it targets only half the muscle groups, per session, of a full-body routine, a two-day split involves a relatively large training volume, which is why I recommend using both moderate resistance (approximately 65 to 75 percent of your SRM) and a moderate repetition range (12 to 15). The two-day split routine may be effectively implemented two or three times a week, provided you alternate upper and lower body training days.

The Three-Day Split

The three-day split further divides the upper body into "push" (extensor) and "pull" (flexor) muscles. This split allows for increased training intensity, or 6 to 15 repetitions at about 70 to 80 percent of your SRM. The three-day split should be implemented as a weekly program to allow for a full week's recovery for each training zone.

The Four-Day Split

The four-day split, as described in Split Routine E, offers the possibility for even greater intensity by adding another work day. However, I would not recommend using split-system E unless your training goals include size and power with little regard for endurance or definition. (These issues will be covered in greater depth in Chapter 7.) The recommended repetition range for this particular split is low, on the order of 3 to 8 repetitions, combined with very heavy weights (80 to 95 percent of your SRM). The recommended exercises include exclusively multijoint power movements, and the recommended recovery for each training zone is ten days.

REVIEW The Ins and Outs of Split Routines

1. A split routine targets a specific zone of the body during each workout and usually hits the entire body over two or three weekly sessions.

2. If you decide to graduate to a split system, start with the split routine that requires roughly the same time commitment as your current full body routine.

3. A two-day split involves a relatively large training volume and should include with moderate resistance and a moderate repetition range of 12 to 15. It may be implemented two or three times a week.

4. The three-day split allows for increased training intensity, of perhaps 6 to 15 repetitions at about 70 to 80 percent of your SRM. It should be implemented weekly.

5. Avoid split routine E unless your specific training goals emphasize both power and muscle size to the exclusion of endurance and definition.

CIRCUIT TRAINING FOR THE TIME-CONSTRAINED

The goal of any resistance work, from circuit programs to powerlifting, is to increase or maintain muscular tone and strength. The main difference between circuit training and most other forms of weight lifting is that it carries an additional objective: to access and remain within the aerobic zone.

Circuit training and heavy weight lifting sit on opposite ends of a wide spectrum of workout techniques. If your weight-lifting program incorporates low repetitions (6 to 15) and moderate to heavy weights (70 to 80 percent of your SRM), the energy demand of your muscles rapidly exceeds your aerobic capacity. Translation: Your cardiovascular system is not equipped to fuel extreme muscular contractions by burning fat. Instead, your muscles rely primarily on anaerobic energy sources. The drawback of always training within the anaerobic zone is that it doesn't burn much fat, nor does it significantly impact cardiovascular stamina.

Circuit training, on the other hand, enables you to remain with the aerobic zone, burning fat while improving cardiovascular health and endurance. The drawback of circuit training is that it builds less muscle and develops only limited explosive strength. If you are a power athlete, such as a sprinter or bodybuilder, you will not reach your full athletic potential exclusively through circuit training. However, if you are an endurance athlete, such as a long-distance runner or cyclist, or if you simply want to tone, firm, and lose weight without bulking up, circuit training might be just what the doctor ordered. And if you're on a tight schedule (who isn't, these days?), properly executed circuit work possesses the advantage of combining cardiovascular training with a weight-lifting session, cutting your total workout time in half.

In order to reap the full benefits of circuit training, you should stay within the target aerobic zone for at least thirty minutes. How can you tell if you're "in the zone"? Simple: Monitor your heart rate. For uninterrupted readings, a heart rate monitor, which can be worn on the wrist or around the chest, is a worthwhile investment. Alternatively, you can use the old-fashioned method and check your pulse.

Most experts agree that exercising between 60 and 70 percent of your maximum heart rate (MHR) places you well within the target zone. In order to calculate your maximum heart rate, subtract your age from the number 220. Multiply this figure by 60 percent and then 70 percent to yield the upper and lower limits of your target zone. A good rule of thumb: If you can whistle a tune, you're probably not going hard enough.

Compared to more strenuous forms of resistance training, circuit work places less stress on your muscles, resulting in less micro-trauma and a shorter recovery period. As a result, you can train the same body part two or three times a week without suffering the ill effects of overtraining. However, if you have never engaged in resistance training or you've taken a significant break from it, start gradually with a very light resistance that allows you to complete the set at the upper range of recommended repetitions (20 to 30).

Proper Technique

Circuit training incorporates higher reps (15 to 30) and lighter weights. In order to reap the full cardiovascular (and fat-burning) benefits of circuit training, you should take little or no rest between sets. However, neglecting rest between sets does not mean you should rush through your workout. As with any other form of resistance exercise, the key to successful, injury-free training is strict attention to form. Review "Use Good Form" on page 95 for more details.

The Machine Circuit

When it comes to circuit training, machines are a great way to minimize injury risk. In addition, because your movements with a machine are somewhat restricted, it is more difficult, but not impossible, to cheat. Perhaps the greatest advantage of machines over free weights during a circuit is that machines are generally faster to adjust to the appropriate resistance. Remember: You have to keep moving to stay in the target zone.

Some gyms provide a series of weight machines located in close proximity specifically for circuit training. If this is not the case at your gym, don't despair. It's easy to design your own circuit (see below).

What if somebody grabs your machine while you're at another point in the circuit? Once you leave a station, the machine is up for grabs. However, most people are happy to accommodate someone who wants to "work in" for a set, especially if you explain that you are completing a circuit. If you run across a jerk who refuses the favor, either jog in place until he's done (this will keep your heart rate elevated, plus it will probably annoy the jerk) or find a free station.

Basic Circuits

When it comes to designing a circuit, the possibilities are virtually endless. Several basic tenets, however, should be kept in mind.

First, you will see the best results if you avoid working the same muscle group two days in a row. The only exceptions to this rule include the abdominal and calf muscles, which many fitness professionals believe you can train daily without suffering ill consequences.

Second, the fewer body parts you include in each session, the more muscular development you will observe in the long run. For example, a 30-minute full-body circuit performed three times a week will probably induce less muscular hypertrophy (growth) than a split system that also requires three 30-minute sessions per week.

Third, as is the case with other weight-training programs, the best way to continue to see excellent results is to make frequent small changes to your routine. Target specific muscle groups with different exercises from week to week; alter your foot stance on presses and squats; change grips on pull-downs and cable rows; go from an upper/lower body split to a push-pull split; experiment. Don't be afraid to try new equipment, movements, or even gyms. And most important, try to have fun!

Appendix C gives three examples of different circuit-training routines. If you've never trained with weights before or have taken an extended break from resistance training, I recommend using the full-body routine for a couple weeks before graduating to either of the splits.

REVIEW Self-Assessment: Is Circuit Training for You?

1. Is your primary objective fat loss rather than strength increase or muscular gain?

2. Is your time extremely limited?

3. With circuit training, toning your body may take longer than with traditional weight-training routines. Do you have the patience?

If you answered "yes" to all of the above questions, circuit training could be your ticket to strong muscles and a healthy cardiovascular system.

Refining Your Routine

I t's time to define your weight-training objectives. Not many would object to improving body aesthetics by sculpting a firm, toned physique. In fact, I think it's safe to assume that for most people, health and aesthetics are top priorities. But what if you participate in sports? Are you a power athlete whose main objective on the field is short bursts of intense, explosive strength? Are you an endurance athlete whose main objective on the field is sustained output? Does your job call for heavy lifting? Or running up and down flights of stairs? Are you a naturally thin person who experiences difficulty gaining weight? Or are you naturally muscular and concerned about becoming too bulky with weight training? Although the basic tenets of weight training are the same for everyone, subtle variations in your workout strategy can make a world of difference to your training outcome.

MUSCLE PHYSIOLOGY FOR THE NONPHYSIOLOGIST

Muscle tissue is composed primarily of two types of fiber: slow-twitch fibers and fast-twitch fibers. The proportion of each fiber in a given sample of muscle tissue depends on a number of factors, the most significant being the type of muscle from which the sample was derived, as well as the particular genetics of the individual from whom the sample was taken. Slow-twitch fibers are distinguishable from fast-twitch fibers by their smaller size and greater endurance capacity. Because slow-twitch fibers fatigue gradually, they are capable of contracting repeatedly for an extended duration. They make the dominant muscular contribution to activities that require extended stamina, such as long-distance cycling and marathon running. Fast-twitch fibers, on the other hand, are more voluminous and possess greater force capacity than their slow-twitch counterparts. Although they are capable of overcoming far greater resistance than slow-twitch fibers are, fast-twitch fibers fatigue after fewer repetitions. They make the dominant contribution to brief power activities, such as sprints and powerlifts.

In a simplified nutshell, you can think of slow-twitch fibers as small endurance fibers and fast-twitch as large strength fibers. Each type of fiber responds best to different training strategies. To build slow-twitch fibers and local endurance, you would use high ranges of repetitions (15 to 20), lighter weights (60 to 70 percent of your single repetition maximum [SRM]), and shorter rest periods (30 to 45 seconds) between sets. Conversely, to build fast-twitch fibers and maximize muscle strength and size, you would use lower ranges of repetitions (3 to 8), heavier weights (80 to 95 percent of your SRM), and longer rest periods (between 2 and 4 minutes) between sets. To evenly stimulate both fiber types, I recommend using a moderate repetition range (6 to 15), a moderate weight range (70 to 80 percent of your SRM) and a moderate rest period of about 60 to 90 seconds.

REVIEW Muscle Physiology

1. Slow-twitch fibers are small endurance fibers. They make the dominant contribution to activities that require extended stamina, such as long-distance cycling and marathon running.

2. Fast-twitch fibers are large strength fibers. They make the dominant contribution to brief power activities, such as sprints and powerlifts.

3. To build slow-twitch fibers and local endurance, use high repetition ranges (15 to 20), lighter weights (60 to 70 percent of your SRM), and short rest periods (30 to 45 seconds) between sets.

4. To build fast-twitch fibers and maximize muscle strength and size, use lower repetition ranges (3 to 8), heavier weights (80 to 95 percent of your SRM), and longer rest periods (up to 2 minutes) between sets.

5. To evenly stimulate both fiber types, use a moderate repetition

range (6 to 15), a moderate weight range (70 to 80 percent of your SRM), and a moderate rest period of about a minute.

TRAINING FOR YOUR AESTHETIC OBJECTIVES

The vast majority of people who own a gym membership engage in weight training primarily for reasons of health and aesthetics. Because most individuals demonstrate a fairly even mix of both slow-twitch and fast-twitch muscle fibers, most physiques respond best to moderate repetition ranges (6 to 15) and moderate resistances (70 to 80 of the SRM), which will target both fiber types. This approach builds strength while also enhancing local endurance. Moreover, this training strategy typically provides the most desirable aesthetic outcome: a lean, toned physique, with firm shapely muscles. The three-day split routines outlined in Appendix C are good examples of this type of moderate-repetition/moderate-resistance strategy.

Don't be afraid to train hard! For the majority of women, the most significant obstacle to the firm, toned physique they strive to possess is the fear of training with intensity. Your muscles will not respond without sufficient stimulation. Muscle takes time to grow. Even if you happen to be one of the very few women blessed with the genetic potential to build big muscles, it doesn't happen overnight. When you are satisfied with the degree of muscularity you have attained, it is very simple to maintain your physique without the slightest risk of ever sprouting huge, unsightly muscles.

When Genetics and Aesthetics Don't Jibe

Although most people tend to exhibit a relatively even mix of the slow-twitch and fast-twitch fibers, somewhere between 5 and 10 percent of people possess a significantly greater quantity of one fiber type.

Mesomorphs have more of the larger fast-twitch fibers. They gain muscle easily. They often look quite muscular even if they don't work out. If they are short in stature, coaches and teammates often marvel at "how strong they are for their size." If they are tall, they are often described as "powerful" or "solid," and they gravitate to defensive positions in team sports. True mesomorphs excel at power sports. They are natural-born sprinters, powerlifters, and shot-putters.

On the other end of the spectrum we find the ectomorphs. Ectomorphs have more of the smaller slow-twitch fibers. They are often described as "skinny" and can have a hard time gaining weight of any kind, muscle or fat. The envy of all their friends, ectomorphs can gorge like starved animals and remain thin. True ectomorphs excel at endurance sports. They are natural-born distance runners, cyclists, and swimmers. Check out any major triathlon and I guarantee the first ones to cross the finish line will be ectomorphs.

Many people have body types that tend toward one end of the spectrum or the other but still do very well with a standard, moderate-strength training routine. If your body type genuinely defies the norms, however, you may need to alter your training strategy to achieve your aesthetic objectives. This is where designing a routine can become complicated!

In the early stages of weight training, regardless of your body type, I advise everyone to follow the general recommendations for the beginner. In other words, start with a high-repetition, full-body program. When you are ready, move on to the split system that best accommodates your lifestyle. If you find that your physique is not responding the way you would like, use what you have learned thus far to refine and personalize your routine to better fit your aesthetic objectives. Some examples are given below.

The Short Mesomorph Who Worries about Stockiness

Given your small frame and propensity for muscular gain, your concerns about bulk are understandable. To prevent stockiness, try training each body part once per week using a high range of repetitions (15 to 20), which will maximally stimulate your slow-twitch fibers. For example, you might use the three-day split described in Appendix C but use a higher number of repetitions and light resistance for each exercise. Likewise, you should become an ardent stretcher. Always stretch before, during, and after your weight-training sessions to prevent tight, short muscles and promote longer, leaner lines.

The Ectomorph Who Can't Seem to Gain Any Muscle

Always train to muscle fatigue. For maximum muscular development, use heavier weights and a lower repetition range, which will preferentially target your fast-twitch muscle fibers. Emphasize multijoint power movements. For example, you might use the three-day split described in Appendix C but substitute power movements for defining movements, using a low repetition range on the order of 6 to 8 per set. You might even try the four-day-split outlined in Appendix C until you begin to notice appreciable gains. Don't be afraid to train with maximum intensity! Train each muscle group past the point of muscle fatigue all the way to failure every second or third workout.

To prevent muscle wasting during your cardiovascular training, don't exceed 60 to 70 percent of your maximum heart rate (MHR). (Remember, to find your maximum heart rate, subtract your age from 220.) Always eat something within an hour after you finish training. This applies to both cardiovascular workouts and weight-training sessions. If you plan to complete your aerobic and resistance training during the same session, start with weight lifting and have an endurance bar or drink and/or a meal replacement bar or drink before you begin the aerobic component of your workout.

REVIEW Four Facts for Sculpting Beauty

1. Most physiques respond best to moderate repetition ranges (6 to 15) with moderate resistances (70 to 80 percent of your SRM).

2. Mesomorphs have more of the larger fast-twitch fibers and gain muscle easily. True mesomorphs *may* need to train with lighter weights and more repetitions to prevent stockiness.

3. Ectomorphs have more of the smaller slow-twitch muscle fibers and have difficulty gaining weight. True ectomorphs *may* need to increase their training intensity and train like a power athlete to make appreciable gains.

4. In the early stages of weight training, regardless of body type, every beginner should adhere to a high-repetition, full-body program.

TRAINING FOR YOUR ATHLETIC OBJECTIVES

When a muscle fiber is stimulated to contract, it will always do so to the greatest possible tension. However, depending on the fiber type, contraction occurs at different rates. Slow-twitch muscle fibers can contract repeatedly every 0.1 seconds without fatiguing, provided sufficient oxygen is available. Fast-twitch fibers develop tension much more rapidly (roughly five times faster than slow-twitch fibers) but fatigue rapidly, regardless of whether or not oxygen is available.

The reason behind these discrepancies becomes apparent when you consider the fact that slow-twitch and fast-twitch fibers exploit vastly different energy schemes. Slow-twitch fibers utilize aerobic (requiring the presence of oxygen) energy production to fuel long-term, submaximal efforts like a 10-kilometer run. Fast-twitch fibers, on the other hand, utilize anaerobic (which does not require oxygen) energy production to fuel short-term, intense efforts like a 100-meter sprint. At the two extremes of aerobic and anaerobic conditioning, we find the endurance athlete and the power athlete, respectively. Through specialized training, each develops her cardiovascular system, aerobic capacity, and muscular responses according to her sport-specific needs.

Weight Training for Agility and Endurance

Resistance training to build agility and stamina should target slow-twitch fibers by employing high repetitions, relatively light weights, and no more than 30 to 45 seconds of rest between sets. If your primary goal is to become a stronger endurance athlete, train at the high end of the range of recommended repetitions (15 to 20 per set) and work each muscle group to fatigue, not failure, once per week. For best results, I recommend using a full-body routine, a full-body circuit routine, or a two-day split routine.

Weight Training for Both Strength and Stamina

Unfortunately, endurance is often gained at the price of strength, and vice versa, depending on which fiber type and energy system dominate the sport-specific training methods. This would not pose a problem if your sport relied entirely on either power or endurance. However, the majority of activities require a dual contribution, combining both power and endurance. Just think of soccer, tennis, hockey, basketball, mountain biking, snowboarding, and rock climbing, to name a few. Moderate-intensity strength training, employing a moderate repetition range (6 to 15) and moderate resistances (70 to 80 percent of your SRM), is appropriate for building the strength *and* stamina most athletic activities require. Fortuitously, this also happens to be the program that produces the best aesthetic results for most body types. For a routine that fits the bill, check out the three-day splits outlined in Appendix C.

If you are serious about athletics, one of the surest ways to guarantee your training covers all bases is to combine some form of prolonged submaximal conditioning with short-term, high-intensity drills. Prolonged submaximal training (at 60 to 80 percent of your MHR) stimulates primarily slow-twitch fibers while also inducing beneficial muscular adaptations that include increased blood flow and energy production from fat sources. High-intensity interval training, on the other hand, stimulates fast-twitch fibers and maximizes cardiovascular output. These physiological events optimize intracellular oxygen availability, help reduce lactic acid accumulation, and promote better performance. As an example of this type of training, once or twice a week, instead of your usual cardiovascular session, you might try running on a track at 60 to 80 percent of your MHR for 45 minutes. Every half mile, do a 100-meter all-out sprint.

Weight Training for Explosive Strength, Power, and Muscularity

If your training objectives include developing explosive power, maximizing strength gains, and becoming as muscular as possible, your training routine should focus on stimulating fast-twitch muscle fibers. Use the fewest number of recommended repetitions (3 to 8) with maximum intensity and heavy weights (80 to 95 percent of your SRM), and rest for 2 to 4 minutes between sets. Emphasize multijoint power movements over defining exercises. Train each body part past muscle fatigue all the way to exhaustion. Take muscle groups to failure once every week to ten days. Refer to the four-day split routine in Appendix C for an example of this type of program.

If you do both weight training and cardiovascular training during the same training session, begin your workout with weights and consume an engineered meal replacement or high-protein/low-carb product before you move on to cardio. To avoid muscle wasting, do not exceed 60 to 70 percent of your maximum heart rate during the cardiovascular component of your training. Have a high-protein meal or engineered product within one hour of completing your workout.

REVIEW Five Facts for Excelling at Athletics

1. Slow-twitch fibers utilize aerobic methods of energy production to fuel long-term, submaximal efforts. Fast-twitch fibers utilize anaerobic methods of energy production to fuel for short-term, intense efforts.

2. Resistance training to build agility and stamina should target slow-twitch fibers with high repetitions (15 to 20), relatively light weights (60 to 70 percent of your SRM), and no more than 30 to 45 seconds of rest between sets. Try either a full-body routine, a full-body circuit routine, or a two-day split.

3. Moderate-intensity strength training, with moderate repetition ranges (6 to 15) using moderate resistances (70 to 80 percent of your SRM), is appropriate for most athletic activities. Try one of the three-day splits outlined in Appendix C.

4. To guarantee that your training enhances both power and endurance, once or twice a week, instead of your usual cardiovascular session, try running on a track at 60 to 80 percent of your MHR for 45 minutes. Every half mile, do a 100-meter, all-out sprint.

5. Resistance training to build explosive power and muscularity should target fast-twitch fibers with low repetitions (3 to 8), heavy weights (80 to 95 percent of your SRM), and at least 2 to 4 minutes of rest between sets. Refer to the four-day split routine in Appendix C for an example of this type of program.

ADVANCED TRAINING TECHNIQUES

As you fall into a comfortable routine, it is sometimes easy to forget one of the most basic tenets of weight training: For optimal muscular development, you must make frequent, subtle changes to your lifting regimen. As you learn to isolate specific muscle groups, your brain ascertains the most efficient way to work against defined directions of resistance. If you are a novice weight lifter, these brain-muscle connections will be well formed after about three weeks of consistent training. As you gain experience, you must find ways to fool your brain into thinking it is doing something new and different. Following the same, monotonous lifting routine month after month will first result in strength plateaus, followed by strength decrements. It's a known fact that tedium frequently leads to overtraining.

When you work against a resistance, your brain signals different muscle groups to fire in a specific order. As you do more repetitions, the first muscle fibers called to perform become fatigued, and new fibers are recruited to the process. Eventually you arrive at muscle fatigue, the point at which you can no longer take the weight through a full range of motion without cheating. Unfortunately, even at muscle fatigue, a significant portion of the muscle has yet to be fully challenged. In general, the only way to ensure that you have hit the entire muscle is to do a number of different exercises that offer different angles and directions of resistance. For optimal muscular growth, I recommend performing at least two different movements for each body part every time you work out. By the same token, you should not restrict yourself to the same two or three exercises week after week. Switch things up to activate the entire muscle.

But what if your workout facility is small and offers only limited exercise alternatives? What if certain movements give you such an incredible pump that you like to do them every time you work a specific muscle group? There are dozens of ways to spice up your workout without having to change the exercises you do. The following methods are just a few of the tried and true. Give them a shot and watch the gains come.

Ascending Sets

Add weight with each consecutive set. If you are training to fatigue with good form, the number of repetitions you are able to do per set will decrease as the load increases. In general, I don't recommend falling below 5 or 6 repetitions, even for the heaviest set.

For Example: After your warm-up set, do your first working set with a relatively light weight; say 60 percent of your SRM. For your second set, jump to 70 percent of your SRM. On your third set, go to 80 percent. For your fourth and final set, try 90 percent. If you are feeling especially strong, go for the gusto with 95 percent of your SRM for your "peak" set.

Descending Sets

After the initial warm-up set, start your first working set with the greatest amount of weight. With successive sets, decrease the weight in increments. Because you are fatiguing the muscle as you go lighter, your repetition range should not change significantly.

For Example: After a solid initial warm-up set, jump directly to 90 percent of your SRM, and take it to the point of muscle fatigue. Drop to 75 percent on your next set. On your third set, drop to 60 percent. For your fourth and final working set, go extra light, say 40 percent of your SRM, and take it to the point of muscle failure.

Pyramid Sets

Pyramids combine the principles of both ascending and descending sets. The weight is first increased with each consecutive set. When you reach the resistance at which you are able to complete only four to six repetitions prior to fatigue, reverse the procedure and decrease the resistance with each consecutive set.

For Example: After your warm-up set, do your first working set with a relatively light weight; say 60 percent of your SRM. For your second set, jump to 70 percent. On your third set (your heaviest set), go to 80 or 90 percent. Drop to 70 percent of your SRM for your fourth set and 50 percent for your fifth and final set.

Super Sets

Rather than taking a break between sets, you can *super-set* by going directly on to a different exercise. Super sets may target one or two muscle groups. (Trying to target more than two groups puts you in the realm of circuit training, which is not the most efficient method for adding muscle mass.) They may also target synergistic muscles (muscles that work together) or antagonistic muscles (muscles that oppose one another). Because you are eliminating the recovery time between sets, super-setting is a great way to streamline your workouts when you are pressed for time. Done properly, super sets are exhausting and require additional concentration. I don't recommend incorporating super sets if you are feeling mentally drained before your workout.

Example 1: Super-Setting Synergistic Muscles. Perform a single light warm-up set for your pectoral muscles and then a light warm-up set for your shoulders. Begin the first round of the super set with the incline press, followed immediately by a set of anterior dumbbell raises to target the anterior head of your deltoid complex. Repeat the working super sets for three additional rounds. When super-setting two exercises that target synergistic muscle groups, you may need to take a brief rest after every second set.

Example 2: Super-Setting Antagonistic Muscles. Start with a light warm-up set for your biceps followed by a light warm-up set for your triceps. Begin the super set with incline dumbbell curls (for biceps) and go immediately to overhead extensions (for triceps). Try completing four rounds of super sets without any breaks. You may need to incorporate descending sets into the routine as you exhaust your arms.

Partial Sets

When sets of partial repetitions are done consecutively, you are actually accomplishing a form of intramuscular (that is, within the same muscle group) super set. Begin your exercise by performing only half of the full range of motion. After five to ten repetitions, move on to just the second half of the motion range. After 5 to 10 repetitions, finish the set with 5 to 10 repetitions of the full range of motion for a total of 20 to 30 repetitions per set.

For Example: After completing a light warm-up set for your biceps, choose a barbell representing 50 to 60 percent of your SRM for standing barbell curls. Begin the set by raising the barbell from the fully extended (elbows straight) position to the point at which your elbows are bent at a 90° angle. The barbell should be just about level with your navel and perpendicular to your body. Perform your first group of repetitions strictly within this abbreviated range. Without releasing the bar, change your motion range two or three repetitions prior to fatigue. Your new starting position is now where your old ending position was, at the point where your elbows are bent at a 90° angle. From here, raise the bar to the fully flexed (elbows maximally bent) position. Again, continue pumping out repetitions until you sense that you are approaching fatigue. For the final phase, lower the bar all the way to the fully extended position, and raise it to the fully flexed position. Perform full-range repetitions all the way to failure. Watch out—it might come sooner than you anticipated!

Strip or Drop Sets

In strip or drop sets, weight is removed or resistance is decreased during the set as muscle fatigue is reached. Strip sets are best accomplished with a partner and are virtually impossible if you are working out alone with free weights. If you normally do several sets of a couple different exercises per muscle group, it would be inadvisable to do strip sets for every set of every exercise. Try strip-setting only as the last set of each exercise. Alternatively, try strip-setting each set of the last exercise only.

For Example: Say you're ready to do the last set of cable rows and you plan for it to be a strip set, with the help of your partner. You begin by using 80 percent of your SRM. After 6 repetitions, you reach fatigue and your partner quickly drops the weight to 60 percent of your SRM. Without missing a beat you rip out 7 more repetitions and again reach fatigue. Your partner drops the weight to 50 percent of your max. After 6 reps you reach fatigue again. Down to 30 percent of your max. This time you can only do 4 reps. Your muscles are completely spent, and now it's your partner's turn.

Any of the advanced training methods described above can be combined. Try strip-setting partial sets, super-setting pyramids, or strip-setting super sets. The possibilities are infinite. One final piece of advice: Experiment! Find what works best for you. Variety is the spice not only of life but also of the gym. Bring variety to your workouts and watch your muscles respond!

REVIEW Advanced Techniques

1. Ascending sets: Add weight with each consecutive set.

2. Descending sets: Decrease weight with each consecutive set.

3. Pyramid sets: Increase weight with each consecutive set. When you reach the resistance at which you are able to complete only 4 to 6 repetitions, decrease the resistance with each consecutive set.

4. Super sets: Rather than taking a break between sets, go directly on to a different exercise that targets the same or a second muscle group.

5. Partial sets: Perform only half of the full range of motion of an exercise. After 5 to 10 repetitions, move on to the second half of the motion range. After an additional 5 to 10 repetitions, finish the set with 5 to 10 repetitions of the full range of motion.

6. Strip or drop sets: Remove weight or decrease resistance during the set as muscle fatigue is reached.

TRAINING SUPPLEMENTS THAT REALLY WORK

Unlike the pharmaceutical industry, the sports supplement industry is largely unregulated. As a result, the consumer is not at the mercy of lobbyists and special interest groups who may or may not profit from the introduction of a new ergogenic substance. We are, however, at the mercy of the supplement companies. Lamentably, the sports supplement industry is notorious for its unscrupulous marketing tactics and cost-cutting manufacturing practices. The consumer is regularly subjected to mountains of misinformation, outlandish claims, and products choked with fillers and contaminants. Disseminating the subterfuge is an ambitious undertaking. What follows is a list of substances that, in my mind, constitute the most effective ergogenic, or performance-enhancing, products available in today's market. Don't risk your health or waste your hard-earned cash by investing in dubious products. Before you spend another cent on supplementation, arm yourself with the knowledge to make an informed decision.

Caffeine

Caffeine is probably the most widely consumed ergogenic, or performance-enhancing, substance known to man. Caffeine acts as a stimulant by virtue of the fact that it is an adenosine antagonist; in other words, it blocks adenosine, a naturally occurring depressant. Caffeine resembles adenosine closely enough to fit into the specific cellular brain receptors that normally accommodate adenosine. By occupying these sites, caffeine prevents adenosine from mediating its depressant effects. Moreover, various studies have demonstrated that caffeine significantly enhances the strength of skeletal muscle and delays the onset of fatigue during endurance exercise. Caffeine also has mild bronchiodilatory effects. For more information on caffeine's thermogenic (fat burning) properties and cautionary statements, please refer to "The Skinny on Fat Burners" on page 51.

Chromium (Chromium Picolinate)

Chromium enables insulin to bind to its receptor sites, facilitating glucose entry for intracellular energy production and promoting amino acid uptake for intracellular protein synthesis. In other words, chromium helps ensure optimal energy levels, muscle recovery, and lean tissue development. Inadequate dietary chromium is believed to contribute to increased fatigue, impaired athletic performance, and suboptimal muscular development. Long-term chromium deficiency may even play a role in the development of cardiovascular disease, high cholesterol levels, obesity, and diabetes. As you may remember from Chapter 4, North Americans are notoriously deficient in chromium. For active individuals, most references recommend chromium supplementation in the form of chromium picolinate to be consumed orally in the amount of 200 to 400 mcg twice daily. For more information on chromium's fat-burning powers, please refer to "The Skinny on Fat Burners" on page 51.

Creatine (Creatine Monohydrate)

Creatine monohydrate exploded onto the fitness scene in 1992. In an industry replete with bogus products and scam supplements, word spread quickly that creatine was the real deal. At the lab and in the gym, creatine induced formidable muscular gains and impressive strength increases. Heralded as the natural alternative to anabolic steroids, creatine's reputation among power athletes flourished. Among today's professional athletes, creatine is the most widely used ergogenic supplement. Fifty percent of National Football League players and at least 25 percent of professional hockey, baseball, and basketball players take creatine. It's rumored that the Los Angeles Lakers keep tubs of it in their locker room. During the 1996 Summer Olympics, three out of four medalists supplemented with creatine. In the second millennium, I predict that you will be hard-pressed to find an Olympic athlete who doesn't use creatine.

If biochemistry lulls you into a coma, you may want to skim through the following long-winded explanation of why creatine represents such a powerful ergogenic substance. You can always come back to this section later should you need further clarification. Just be aware of the following: Creatine is probably the safest, most effective nonhormonal agent you can take to significantly increase muscle mass, strength, power, and stamina. Even if you never try another training supplement, consider giving creatine monohydrate a test drive. You won't regret it.

How Does Creatine Work?

Creatine is a nonessential amino acid found in high abundance in muscle meats and fish. A pound of red meat, salmon, or tuna contains approximately 2 grams of creatine. Creatine can either be absorbed from the diet or synthesized in the liver and pancreas from its precursor amino acids glycine, arginine, and methionine. When creatine enters the circulation, it is delivered to skeletal muscle, where it undergoes an enzymatic reaction involving the attachment of a high-energy phosphate group to yield phosphocreatine (PC). Phosphocreatine, in turn, donates the phosphate group necessary to generate the high-energy molecule adenosine tri-phosphate (ATP) from its low-energy form, adenosine di-phosphate (ADP). ATP is the fuel our bodies utilize for most intracellular reactions, including the contraction of muscle fibers. Because stores of ATP are limited, our ability to perform at maximal effort is directly related to the availability of PC, which itself is directly related to the availability of raw creatine. Concentrations of intramuscular PC affect both the magnitude and duration of energy generated during intense exercise. As PC depletes, so does performance.

Without supplementation, the human body normally stores between 120 and 160 grams of creatine, both free and phosphorylated (in the form of PC). Ninety-five percent of these creatine stores are found in muscle tissue. Acute creatine loading (20 grams per day for seven days) has been shown to increase intramuscular concentrations of creatine by up to 40 percent. Following the loading phase, enhanced creatine reservoirs can be maintained by supplementing with 2 to 5 grams of creatine per day. By providing added fuel for muscular contraction, increased creatine stores permit longer, more intense workouts. In addition, there is evidence that greater PC availability augments the rate of ATP generation during and immediately following high-intensity, short-duration efforts, such as weight lifting. Moreover, creatine could potentially prove to increase the buffering mechanisms within working muscle, lessening the impact of lactic acid buildup.

Regardless of what further scientific investigation might reveal, numerous well-documented studies have already confirmed that oral creatine supplementation, in appropriate dosages, over time causes significant increases in strength, power, endurance, work capacity, muscle mass, muscle recovery, athletic performance, and training adaptation. In addition, creatine supplementation has been shown to contribute to a decrease in body fat stores. Creatine also causes a cell-voluminizing phenomenon that has been linked to increased protein synthesis, decreased muscle catabolism, and increased glycogen synthesis. Why, then, is this ubiquitous amino acid still surrounded by controversy?

Be an Informed Consumer: Avoid Counterfeit Creatine!

There are more scam products on the market than legitimate items. For example, liquid creatine was developed based on the premise that a soluble formulation would permit faster, more complete absorption into systemic circulation. Unfortunately, two basic flaws are inherent to this logic. First, creatine monohydrate is already absorbed at rates approaching 100 percent. The challenge confronting scientists and manufacturers has not been to get the creatine from the digestive tract into the bloodstream but, rather, to get the creatine from the bloodstream into muscle cells. In addition, liquid creatine begins to degrade after only a few days, producing creatinine, a harmless but useless byproduct of creatine metabolism. Because there is no way for a consumer to determine how long liquid creatine has been sitting on the shelf, it's difficult to establish its viability.

Creatine monohydrate plus citric acid and potassium carbonate equals effervescent creatine. Like liquid creatine, effervescent creatine was developed based on the premise that increased solubility would lead to increased absorption. As outlined above, creatine monohydrate is already well absorbed into the circulation. According to scientific investigation, effervescent creatine is no better at getting into muscle cells than its fizzless counterpart. On the other hand, effervescent creatine is better at getting into your wallet and extracting greater sums of revenue.

With the current state of technology, straight creatine monohydrate in powder form is still the only way to go. However, creatine powder alone is not enough. Studies demonstrate that a significant insulin spike is necessary to initiate the mechanism that drives creatine into skeletal muscle. Hence, in order for your muscles to benefit from creatine supplementation, you must also consume a sizable dose of high-glycemic-index (HGI) carbohydrates. In the past, bodybuilders have attempted to potentiate creatine delivery by taking their creatine with grape juice. Unfortunately, grape juice is largely comprised of low-glycemic-index (LGI) fructose, or fruit sugar, which is incapable of generating a substantial insulin spike. Nowadays, you can find creatine monohydrate preparations that contain enough dextrose (or a similar HGI sugar) to ensure expedient creatine shuttling into skeletal muscle. For best results, choose a creatine product that contains 75 grams of dextrose per serving.

Ephedrine

Ephedrine works primarily through the release of excitatory chemicals called catecholamines. The catecholamines, which include adrenaline, are responsible for increasing heart rate and peripheral circulation, dilating bronchioles, and raising alertness. The combined effects of ephedrine allow you to increase both your training intensity and the duration of your workout.

On the negative side, ephedrine does demonstrate a low incidence of potentially dangerous side effects. Please refer to "The Skinny on Fat Burners" on page 51 for a list of medical contraindications.

Ephedrine, Caffeine, and Aspirin (ECA) Stack

Some of the most effective ergogenic products contain a synergistic blend of ephedrine, caffeine, and salicylic acid, or aspirin. When these three compounds are stacked, their combined effect tends to be greater than the sum of the individual effects. Caffeine and ephedrine pave the way for heightened alertness, increased heart rate, increased blood flow to skeletal muscles, bronchodilation, enhanced strength of skeletal muscles, and increased stamina during endurance activities. Aspirin (or its herbal equivalent, white willow bark) blocks the body's production of prostaglandins, prolonging these effects. Please refer back to "The Skinny on Fat Burners" on page 51 for a detailed account of the ECA stack as it pertains to fat loss.

Glucosamine Sulfate

Although scientists have not yet proven its mechanism of action, glucosamine sulfate is believed to stimulate the manufacture of glucosaminoglycans, which are key structural components of cartilage. Because cartilage has a poor blood supply, it does not have the capacity to heal itself to the degree that other tissues, such as skin and bone, can. Researchers hypothesize that the increase of glucosaminoglycans stimulated by glucosamine sulfate allows cartilage a greater degree of self-maintenance and repair. In a landmark Belgian study, 500 mg of glucosamine sulfate administered three times daily was shown not only to relieve osteoarthritis pain of the knee, but also to improve joint function and retard progressive destruction of articular cartilage. Results of the investigation may even indicate that glucosamine sulfate is the first orally administered substance with the ability to stimulate cartilage regeneration!

Eighty percent of adults over age fifty suffer from some degree of osteoarthritis. Many athletes, even young athletes, experience degenerative changes as a result of injury. Whereas nonsteroidal anti-inflammatory drugs (NSAIDs) such as aspirin and ibuprofen offer temporary relief from arthritis pain, the improvement in joint function and potential restoration of joint architecture are unique to supplements like glucosamine sulfate. Moreover, long-term glucosamine administration exhibits none of the potentially dangerous side-effects of NSAIDs. But this begs the question: Given the high likelihood that you will eventually develop osteoarthritis in one or more weight-bearing joints (especially if you're athletic), is it possible to prevent the onset of degenerative changes with glucosamine supplementation? Although this notion has not yet been scientifically tested, it makes sense. Perhaps one way to ensure a lifetime of healthy joints and pain-free mobility is to start taking glucosamine sulfate at an early age, before cartilage damage becomes symptomatic.

The currently recommended dosage for the treatment of arthritis pain is 500 mg of glucosamine sulfate taken three times a day. The effects are gradual, and a month or more may pass before you notice marked improvement.

Glucosamine is a natural substance derived from shrimp, lobster, and crab shells and has few contraindications. However, diabetics and those with known shellfish allergies should consult their health care provider before trying it.

Glutamine

Glutamine is the most prevalent amino acid in the human body. Found in abundance in both muscle and plasma, glutamine accounts for more than 60 percent of the free amino acid pool in muscle cells and is crucial to muscle metabolism. Glutamine is best known for its capacity to prevent muscle wasting and help eliminate toxins from the body. Often referred to as the "brain fuel of amino acids," glutamine can move directly from the bloodstream into the central nervous system, providing your brain with glucose substrates when glucose itself is scarce. Glutamine is also essential for rapidly dividing cells like lymphocytes, which play a key role in immune system function.

Many stressors, including physical exertion, can overcome the body's ability to manufacture sufficient glutamine for optimal health and performance. For this reason, glutamine is often referred to as "conditionally essential." During periods of intense training, many athletes take supplemental glutamine to prevent protein catabolism, boost immune function, and avoid symptoms of overtraining.

Whey Protein Isolates

Whey protein isolates (WPIs) are more than 90 percent pure protein and have the highest bioavailability of any known protein source, supporting unparalleled muscle growth and repair. Moreover, whey protein boasts an extremely high concentration of essential amino acids and the highest concentration of branched-chain amino acids (BCAAs) of any single protein source. Studies demonstrate that increased BCAA intake not only improves endurance but also permits muscle sparing during intense training.

For more information on WPIs' role in immune health, see "The Informed Consumer's Guide to Engineered Proteins" on page 25.

REVIEW Effective Ergogenics

1. Caffeine. Caffeine increases alertness, significantly enhances the

How a Mesomorph Bodybuilder Became a Slim, Toned, Physique Model

This is my own personal story. In the summer of 1997, I made a decision that led to a discovery. And the discovery led to a revelation. And the revelation eventually made way for a life-altering epiphany. But I'm getting ahead of myself here. You see, in August 1997, I made the decision to retire from competitive bodybuilding, permanently. At a height of 5'5", I weighed a very muscular 142 pounds and was also faced with the harsh realization that my size was actually impeding my career as an actor, physique model, and fitness personality. Of course my biggest fear (aside from the trepidation of watching all that hard-earned muscle wither away) was that I would get flabby if I significantly decreased the amount that I trained. I began cutting back gradually. I went from a four-day split to a three-day split. I cut my weight training from 12 sets per muscle group to 8 sets. I trained to muscle fatigue instead of muscle failure. I cut my training time from 60 to 30 minutes. I increased my repetition range from 6 to 10 heavy reps to 15 to 20 lighter ones. I maintained my cardio-vascular routine: 45 minutes, five times a week, on the treadmill or stationary bike. Alas, six months later, I'd *gained* more muscle! I topped the scales at a lean and strapping 145 pounds.

Hence the discovery: For years, I had been overtraining. I first started weight lifting when I was a college junior in order to increase my explosive strength and become a more formidable soccer and ice hockey player. I learned the iron ropes from a couple of football-player friends who talked the coach into allowing me to use the varsity weight room after hours. When I went on to medical school, I continued to train with guys. But not just any guys—only the certified muscleheads could keep up with me. When I relocated to Los Angeles after graduating from medical school, I continued to train with men, many of them professional body-builders. At each step, my training became more and more intense, and my training partners used more and more "training aids" (the code word for illegal supplementation). I did not. But it never occurred to me that, as a natural athlete, the amount I was training exceeded my body's capacity to recover. Before I cut back on my weight training, I was constantly sore, regularly fatigued, and frequently ill. Hence the revelation: Three weekly

45- to 60-minute sessions of intense resistance training is the maximum training volume for natural athletes. But back to my story . . .

After six months without appreciable shrinkage, I knew it was time to implement more drastic measures. With a heavy heart, I decided to take an indefinite break from weight training. Still, I maintained my cardiovascular schedule, schlepping into Gold's Gym Venice five times a week to go running and biking to absolutely no destination whatsoever for 45 endless minutes. I ought to mention here that throughout my years of weight lifting, I truly enjoyed the process. My body responded quickly, and I relished in the fact that I was just as strong as most men my size. Cardiovascular workouts, on the other hand, had never been something that I looked forward to. I'd always regarded them as a necessary evil. Now that cardiovascular training was the sole reason I went to the gym, I grew to despise those boring hours spent running and biking in place. For the first time since I was a teenager, I let my gym membership lapse. It seemed like a waste of time and money to drag myself to the gym five times a week when there was a perfectly good track only a few blocks from my apartment. After a couple weeks of running circles around the high school, I hauled my mountain bike out of storage. I hadn't ridden it since medical school, which, incidentally, was also the last time I'd played soccer or hockey—the very reasons I'd started to lift weights in the first place. I got the bike tuned and started exploring the local trails. The fresh air, panoramic views, and aerobic challenge made me look forward to my bike rides more than I'd ever looked forward to going to the gym. In a matter of weeks, I was leaner than I'd ever been during the bodybuilding off-season, and my lungs were stronger than they'd felt in years.

That winter, I got myself a snowboard and started to hit the local mountains. I became so completely addicted to the sport that I began to structure my entire schedule around long weekends spent riding Mammoth Mountain. Toward the end of the ski season, I dusted off my hockey gear and started playing pickup roller hockey. When the ocean warmed up for summer, I borrowed a surf board from my best friend and started to teach myself to surf. After a year of being gym-free, I'd managed to lose about 15 pounds, and I was in the best cardiovascular shape of my entire life. And my physique? Believe it or not, all the cross training had provided the perfect stimuli for reshaping a balanced musculature. I was in the greatest demand of my fitness career and landed a lucrative contract with a leading supplement company shortly thereafter.

When I go to the gym now, I train like an endurance athlete. The high-rep, light-resistance approach is just what my muscles need to stay firm and toned without gaining bulk. In addition, by training to improve my genetic weaknesses (a lack of endurance fibers combined with exercise-induced asthma), I have managed to significantly improve my athletic performance in all areas. I have the strength, endurance, and stamina to mountain bike, snowboard, ski, or surf for literally hours at a time five or six days a week. Moreover, I have become both an expert freestyle snowboarder and proficient downhill mountain biker. I may never again flex my competitive muscles on stage, but I just might try a little racing . . .

Oh, about the revelation that made way for that life-altering epiphany I mentioned earlier—more on that in Chapter 8!

strength of skeletal muscle, and delays the onset of fatigue during endurance exercise. It also has fat-burning properties.

2. **Chromium.** Inadequate dietary chromium can contribute to fatigue, impair athletic performance, and inhibit muscular development.

3. **Creatine.** Oral supplementation with creatine monohydrate results in significant increases in strength, work capacity, muscle mass, muscle recovery, athletic performance, and training adaptation over time. In addition, creatine supplementation has actually been shown to contribute to a decrease in body fat stores.

4. **Ephedrine.** Ephedrine stimulates blood flow to skeletal muscles, increases heart rate, dilates bronchioles, and heightens alertness. Ephedrine is also a highly effective thermogenic fat burner.

5. **Ephedrine, caffeine, and aspirin (ECA) stack.** The ECA stack produces heightened alertness, increased heart rate, increased blood flow to skeletal muscles, bronchodilation, enhanced strength of skeletal muscles, and increased stamina during endurance activities.

6. **Glucosamine sulfate.** Supplementing with glucosamine sulfate

decreases arthritis pain, improves joint function, and retards progressive destruction of articular cartilage.

7. **Glutamine.** This amino acid is best known for its capacity to prevent muscle wasting and eliminate toxins from the body.

8. **Whey protein isolates.** WPIs are high in protein and support muscle growth and repair. They also have a high concentration of essential amino acids and branched-chain amino acids, which improve endurance and permit muscle sparing during intense training.

The Happy, Healthy Approach to Exercise

Most people exercise to achieve optimal health and a beautiful body. Unfortunately, there are a multitude of misconceptions about exercise that—if you buy into them—can make it impossible to achieve either. In fact, some unsound exercise practices are not just ineffective, they're downright dangerous. The objective of this chapter is to help you recognize exercise pitfalls, properly address injury, and avoid overtraining. With a little common sense and knowledge, you can enjoy a lifetime of safe, fun, and effective physical activity.

YOU ARE NOW ENTERING THE AEROBIC ZONE

In reading thus far, you've encountered numerous references pertaining to the importance of aerobic exercise for cardiovascular health and overall longevity. However, until now I have provided very little in the way of specifics about cardiovascular exercise. There's a simple reason for this: Cardio, as it's known, isn't rocket science. Virtually anyone who can move her arms or legs can engage in cardiovascular training. There are, however, a few things you should know to maximize the effectiveness of your training.

Debunking the Myth of Spot Reduction

Fat accumulates on your body in a pattern that is almost completely determined by a combination of genetic factors, sex, and age. Men commonly experience weight gain first around the waist, resulting in the typical apple-shaped body type, complete with love handles and a potbelly. Women, on the other hand, are more prone to add weight first on their hips and thighs, developing a pear-shaped body type. Post-menopausally, a woman's adipose (fat) tissue tends to redistribute toward her waistline, transforming her body type from a pear to an apple. Why bother with these fruity appellations? They may seem a bit silly, but in terms of heart health, your body type plays a significant role in predicting future morbidity. A number of clinical studies have demonstrated that being pear-shaped is much preferable to being apple-shaped. Fat accumulation on the chest and torso is far more likely to occur in association with cardiovascular disease than fat deposits on the hips, thighs, and buttocks. (Of course, the healthiest body type does not reflect an accumulation of fat.)

Contrary to popular misconception, there is no such thing as "spot reduction." In other words, you cannot target a particular area for fat loss. Triceps extensions and other forms of upper-body weight training will not burn the flab off your arms any more than doing lunges will burn it off your hips. Instead, you will ordinarily lose body fat in the reverse order that you put it on.

What Are the Best Forms of Cardiovascular Training?

My answer is very simple: Pick an activity that you can tolerate well enough to do consistently. Your heart doesn't care what you do so long as you do it. Physiologically, your heart can't tell the difference between cycling, stair climbing, or running on a treadmill. All your heart knows is that your muscles are experiencing increased oxygen demands and it must beat faster in order to meet them. The best cardiovascular program is one that is convenient and painless enough to adhere to.

Be aware that certain exercises place more stress on your joints than others. If you suffer from bad knees or a bad back, stick with activities that are low impact. As a general rule, if your feet never leave the surface of the exercise equipment, the activity is probably low impact. For example, while stair running is very high impact, stepping on the stair climber is very low. If your exercise of choice is running, you can reduce the risk of developing shin splints and knee and ankle problems by investing in a good pair of running shoes with plenty of ankle support and a cushioned sole. Also, avoid running on asphalt if you can help it. Tracks, dirt, sand, and grass are all less stressful on your joints.

How Often, and How Long?

Several recent studies have drawn the same conclusion: Men and women who are most successful at losing weight and maintaining weight loss over the long term burn approximately 2,800 calories per week through physical activity. This figure is twice the amount typically recommended for good health and weight control. In order to burn 2,800 calories a week, the average person would have to walk between 25 and 28 miles per week. This translates to walking for about an hour every day. Obviously, participating in more intense activities like swimming or running burns the same number of calories in less time. However, after a certain point, increasing your exercise intensity provides diminishing returns in terms of fat burning.

Surprisingly, low- to moderate-intensity activities are ideal for fat burning. "Low to moderate" corresponds to an exercise intensity that causes your heart to beat at approximately 60 to 70 percent of your maximum heart rate (MHR). To calculate this range and determine your target aerobic zone (TAZ), first subtract your age from the number 220 to estimate MHR. Then multiply this figure by 60 and 70 percent. The two values generated represent the lower and upper limits of your TAZ in beats per minute. For example, a thirty-five-year-old woman would have a target aerobic zone of:

$$
\begin{aligned}
\text{TAZ} &= (\text{MHR} \times 0.6) \text{ to } (\text{MHR} \times 0.7) \\
&= ([220 - 35] \times 0.6) \text{ to } ([220 - 35] \times 0.7) \\
&= (185 \times 0.6) \text{ to } (185 \times 0.7) \\
&= \textbf{111 to 130 beats per minute}
\end{aligned}
$$

In other words, for the average thirty-five-year-old woman, exercising at an intensity that causes her heart to beat between 111 and 130 times per minute is optimal for fat burning. At this exercise intensity, enough oxygen is present to metabolize both carbohydrates and fat in roughly equal proportions. Because it takes more oxygen to metabolize fat than it does carbohydrates, at higher intensities very little fat is burned. At these higher intensities, the body shifts from primarily aerobic (requiring oxygen) to anaerobic (no oxygen necessary) metabolism. High-intensity anaerobic activities include sprints, short-duration power activities like the long jump, and weight training. I can hear what you're thinking: Why, then, should I bother with weight training? The answer is simple: to build muscle. Toned muscle looks fantastic and, in the long run, because it is so highly metabolically active, will help your body consume more calories on a daily basis.

Which Should Come First: Weights or Cardio?

It generally takes about 30 minutes of cardiovascular activity performed within the target aerobic zone to deplete muscle glycogen stores and start burning significant fat. If you plan to do both your aerobic and weight training during the same session, start with the weights. Then your glycogen will be depleted by the time you get to cardio. Theoretically, structuring your workout in this order will cause you to burn maximum fat with minimal concomitant muscle wasting.

The exception to this rule is when you plan to exercise first thing in the morning. In that case, if you intend to do both cardiovascular and strength training, do the cardio first, on an empty stomach. Because your muscles are already depleted of glycogen after a night's sleep, aerobic exercise done first thing in the morning, prior to eating but after a cup of coffee (see "The Skinny on Fat Burners" on page 51), burns more fat than at any other time of day. However, I do not advise that you go straight from empty-stomach cardiovascular exercise to resistance training. By the time you've completed the cardiovascular component of your workout, your body is depleted of glycogen. Resistance training requires glucose. If glucose is not readily available as either muscle glycogen or blood glucose, your body will break down, or catabolize, muscle tissue. Obviously, this process is counterproductive to lean tissue development and muscle toning. Hence, you should always have something to eat between cardiovascular exercise on an empty stomach followed by strength training. An engineered meal replacement is a convenient choice.

REVIEW Solving the Cardio Conundrum

1. You cannot target a problem area with exercise. Only through a sensible combination of diet and cardiovascular activity will you shed fat.

2. The best forms of cardiovascular exercise are whatever activities you can tolerate well enough to do consistently.

3. For successful weight loss and a healthy heart, spend approximately 40 to 60 minutes four or five times per week engaged in aerobic activity.

4. Cardiovascular activity performed within your target aerobic zone (60 to 70 percent of your MHR) is the most efficient means to burn fat.

5. If you do your cardiovascular exercise first thing in the morning on an empty stomach, have a meal replacement before moving on to weight training.

7. With the exception of early morning exercise on an empty stomach, if you plan to do cardiovascular and weight training in the same session, start with the weights.

SURVIVING STRAINS AND SPRAINS

Tendons and ligaments are like springs; when overstretched, they become damaged and will not recoil fully. Ligaments, in particular, are relatively avascular structures (in other words, they have a poor blood supply). They heal badly and often don't return to their original length or strength following an injury. Individuals who have suffered a seriously sprained ankle will attest to the ease with which reinjury occurs. With the common inversion sprain, in which the lateral (outer) part of the foot turns under, permanent ligamentous laxity may result on that side of the ankle. A vicious cycle begins: With each repeated sprain, the ligaments become more stretched, the ankle becomes increasingly unstable, and the likelihood of reinjury escalates.

Immediately following trauma, injured tissue becomes inflamed. The inflammatory response prepares the area for healing and repair by disposing of devitalized tissue. Acute inflammation involves vasodilatation (dilated blood vessels) and increased vascular permeability (leaky blood vessels). These processes cause local heat, redness, swelling, and an influx of white blood cells that functions to clear away cellular debris.

Initial care of a sprain should include nonsteroidal anti-inflammatory agents, ice, rest, elevation, and immobilization with either a cast, taping, or splinting. Nonsteroidal anti-inflammatory drugs such as ibuprofen and naproxen will decrease the pain and swelling associated with the inflammatory process. Acetaminophen, found in Tylenol, will relieve pain but not swelling. Avoid aspirin during the acute phase of injury because it can exacerbate bleeding and hematoma formation.

In order to decrease the vasodilatation that causes edema (swelling caused by excess fluid), cold compresses should be applied for 15 to 20 minutes every two or three hours for the first two days following such an injury. Do not apply heat during the initial stages of inflammation; it will only make the swelling worse.

Most important, be aware that immobilization without rest is not really immobilization. Even with the affected limb in a cast, muscle contraction will propagate blood flow to the injured tissue, causing increased pain and swelling and delaying the healing process.

CAUTION

If significant swelling or discoloration occur in conjunction with obvious deformity, incapacitating pain, loss of sensation, or loss of pulse in the affected limb, see a doctor immediately!

REVIEW Treating a Soft Tissue Injury

1. Initial care of soft tissue injury should include nonsteroidal anti-inflammatory agents, ice, rest, elevation, and immobilization.

2. Avoid aspirin during the acute phase of injury.

3. Administer only cold compresses for the first two days following a soft tissue injury.

HOW TO AVOID OVERTRAINING

So you want to be a better athlete. You want to run farther, sprint faster, throw the ball harder, and push bigger weights. You know that higher levels of conditioning demand physiological challenges, and you are prepared to meet them. You throw yourself into your training with unprecedented fervor. Greater cardiac stroke volume, increased lung capacity, capillary proliferation, muscle fiber hypertrophy—it's all yours for the taking . . . If only it were that simple. Unfortunately, a fine line exists between an effectively progressive exercise regimen that challenges the muscular and cardiovascular systems and one that results in physical burnout. While it's true that increased training loads are necessary for enhanced athletic performance, you must never forget that increased training loads require increased recovery time. If you fail to provide your body with sufficient renewal opportunities, your performance will first taper off, then plateau, and eventually decline.

Overtraining is probably the most common and preventable of all sports injuries. *Overtraining syndrome* is defined as the collection of emotional, behavioral, and physiological sequelae associated with excessive training volume and intensity, which over time accumulate to produce decrements in strength, speed, explosiveness, endurance, and skilled motor performance. The clinical features of overtraining are both diverse and abundant. Common emotional symptoms include altered mood, insomnia, loss of interest, nervousness, and depression. Peripheral features include chronic joint stiffness, overuse injuries, and persistent soreness. And systemic signs can encompass everything from increased incidence of illness to chronic fatigue, loss of appetite, and digestive problems.

As with all health-related issues, prevention is the key to protection. To prevent overtraining, all you need is a modicum of common sense and a training journal. Maintaining a brief, written record of your workouts is an excellent way to both chart your progress and track the intensity and duration of your training sessions. It is also important to monitor the quality of your workout. Increased muscle soreness, deleterious changes in your mood, falling energy levels, or declines in overall performance that persist for more than two weeks probably signal the onset of overtraining. To help prevent boredom and staleness, frequently vary your training methods. Likewise, use a variety of exercises to help avoid monotony. To help prevent overuse injuries, concentrate on using proper form. In addition, set aside at least one day per week for complete relaxation—no weights, no cardio, no significant physical exertion of any kind.

A healthy diet is one of the most powerful weapons in your arsenal against burnout. Although excessive carbohydrate ingestion neither increases muscle glycogen stores nor confers protection against the onset of overtraining (you just get fat), *adequate* carbohydrate ingestion is a critical factor in maximizing both muscle glycogen levels and training tolerance. Consuming sufficient protein is also important. Regardless of the sport, rigorous exercise results in micro-tears within muscle tissue. "Sprint"-type sports, contact sports, and weight training lead to especially large degrees of muscular break-down. Lacking sufficient protein intake, these tissues will neither recover fully nor develop optimally. (See Chapter 2 for more information about healthy dieting.)

The timing of your meals is as crucial as their content. You should have a meal or engineered meal replacement every two to three hours. In addition, you should always have a meal or meal replacement within an hour after you train. Remember, it takes time for digested nutrients to reach exhausted tissues. During the interim, with glycogen stores depleted, your hypoglycemic system will feed off the very muscle you are laboring to build.

Given its significant psychological component, the prevention of overtraining also calls for a concerted effort to avoid undue stress. Make a commitment to yourself to practice stress reduction and get adequate rest. The importance of sleep may seem obvious, but most people still don't get enough. Experts recommend seven to eight hours of sleep per night for increased longevity, decreased stress, and enhanced feelings of well-being. Research demonstrates un-equivocally that adequate sleep is integral to producing improved physical function and mental status.

Finally, listen to your body! If you find you are losing enthusiasm for your workouts, if you are constantly tired, or if your progress has slowed or stopped, it's time for a break. Mild overtraining responds well to three to five days of *complete* rest. Workouts can then be resumed on an alternate-day basis. In more prolonged and severe cases of burnout, the training program may require several weeks of interruption. In such instances, engage in low-intensity activity to help prevent exercise withdrawal and muscle wasting.

REVIEW Don't Overlook Overtraining

1. Monitor the quality of your workouts by noting increased muscle soreness, mood swings, falling energy levels, or declines in overall performance.

2. To prevent boredom and staleness, frequently vary your training methods and use a variety of exercises.

3. To prevent overuse injuries, use proper form and set aside one day a week for complete relaxation.

4. Always eat a high-protein meal within an hour after you train, and make sure your diet includes adequate amounts of proteins and carbohydrates.

5. Get seven to eight hours of sleep per night.

6. If you have overtrained, take three to five days of complete rest before restarting your exercise routine.

BEWARE THE SPECTER OF EXERCISE ADDICTION

Despite all the wonderfully fulfilling aspects of physical activity, a staggering number of men and women struggle with an unhealthy attitude toward exercise. Current estimates indicate that somewhere between 3 and 5 percent of people who exercise regularly engage in dangerous training patterns. The majority of exercise abusers are female, and mental health professionals believe that their numbers are climbing.

Exercise addiction, also referred to as compulsive exercising, exercise bulimia, and activity anorexia, is a recently described phenomenon. It is not yet recognized by the medical community as a diagnostic entity. Hence, it does not receive the kind of attention devoted to more conventional compulsions like overeating, though its consequences can be just as devastating. It was not until 1979 that sports scientists even considered the possibility that exercise could represent a negative compulsion, or even an addiction. Professionals have since conceded that, as is true with any compulsive or addictive behavior, exercise addiction puts the victim's physical and mental health in jeopardy.

For the exercise addict, athletic training comes to take precedence over every aspect of the individual's life. She becomes so dependent on her workouts that she cannot and will not stop, regardless of the cost to physical health, emotional well-being, family, and work. She may ignore other responsibilities that could interfere with her training. She is blind to the fact that she routinely performs far short of her potential because she is perpetually overtrained. Ironically, because exercise is deemed a healthy activity, compulsive exercising often goes unnoticed, or worse still, victims receive encouragement from their peers for their dedication and drive.

For the sake of cardiovascular health, the average individual receives maximum benefits from expending between 2,000 and 3,500 calories per week engaged in low to moderate intensity aerobic activity. This translates to roughly 45 to 60 minutes of exercise four or five times a week. Beyond this, the rewards of aerobic training diminish rapidly until gains are replaced by losses in the form of injuries, illness, exhaustion, decreased productivity, anxiety, and depression.

The Roots of Exercise Addiction

According to Dr. Richard Rosen, Assistant Clinical Professor of Psychiatry at UCLA, exercise addiction probably is one manifestation of the spectrum of symptomatologies that comprise obsessive-compulsive disorder, obsessive personality disorder, or an eating disorder. It may be some time before exercise addiction has been sufficiently mulled over by the medical establishment for proper classification, and probably even longer before mental health experts put forth a working hypothesis as to its etiology. According to sociologists, we live in an age of narcissistic self-absorption. Men and women alike feel the pressure to achieve the ultimate physique: strong, lean, muscular, and aesthetically appealing. Lamentably, it seems the closer we approach this ideal, the more we notice our remaining flaws.

Researchers in the 1980s often suggested that the body's release of endorphins (our natural opiates) could cause an addiction to activities like running. However, a large volume of more recent work has essentially negated this theory. At this point in time, no single, unifying explanation can explain the development of exercise addiction. Many factors are believed to contribute to its genesis. Negative body image, obsessive-compulsive tendencies, low self esteem, and control issues have all been implicated. Like victims of eating disorders, compulsive exercisers often feel overwhelmed by day-to-day demands. For these individuals, exercise provides a sense of control over some aspect of an otherwise chaotic existence. Researchers have, in fact, repeatedly demonstrated that exercise addiction and eating disorders often go hand in hand.

Many experts assert that exercise addiction is a form of eating disorder. Both compulsive exercisers and those who suffer from anorexia and bulimia commonly experience shame, anger, and denial when confronted with their behaviors. Most exercise addicts, like victims of eating disorders, deny their condition for months or years before even considering that they might have a problem.

The Female Athlete Triad

Certain groups of athletes are historically more vulnerable to disordered eating and exercise patterns. Dancers, runners, gymnasts, bodybuilders, and wrestlers are at an elevated risk for serious injury and even death, secondary to their repeated efforts to rapidly shed weight prior to an athletic competition or event. Since fitness competitors also fit this profile, I have little doubt that they will soon be joining the ranks. In fact, current demographics seem to indicate that young, female athletes are at the greatest risk for exhibiting compulsive exercise habits.

The increasingly prevalent combination of irregular menstrual cycles, disordered eating, and osteoporotic bone changes in young women has earned the title "female athlete triad." Many of the young women who suffer from the female athlete triad are exercise addicts.

Disquieting research performed at UCLA has demonstrated that an increasing number of young female athletes are experiencing osteoporotic bone loss. Some of the subjects in the study had, in their early twenties, bone densities comparable to women in their seventies! UCLA researchers blamed these results on the proliferation of compulsive exercising, eating disorders, and the use of steroid for performance enhancement. This deadly blend has female athletes eroding the very bone they will need to last throughout their adulthood.

Extremely low body fat translates to alterations in estrogen metabolism that predisposes women to the development of osteoporosis. It also causes hypothalamic dysfunction, which can result in inadequate stimulation of the ovaries to cause ovulation. When a woman becomes anovulatory (ovulation ceases), her body will not undergo the cyclic production of progesterone that allows for normal menses. Eventually, she may become amenorrheaic (periods cease

Symptoms That May Signal Unhealthy Exercise Habits

- Repeated exercising beyond the requirements for good health.
- Training despite injury.
- Training that takes precedence over work or school responsibilities.
- Exercising at the expense of friendships and relationships.
- Fanaticism about weight, body composition, and diet.
- Performing additional exercise as a "punishment" for eating too much.
- Canceling appointments in order to make more time for exercise.
- A predilection for thinking and talking exclusively about exercise.
- Keeping scrupulously detailed diet and training records.
- A tendency to define one's self-worth in terms of performance.
- A tendency to define one's self-worth in terms of body composition.
- An absence of a sense of accomplishment regarding athletic achievements.
- A perpetual dissatisfaction with one's body image.
- A lack of ability to savor victories.
- An inclination to focus entirely on the challenge of exercise.
- A lack of enjoyment for the training process.
- Suffering from exercise withdrawal when activities are impossible.
- Feelings of guilt or anxiety when workouts are missed.
- Frequent injuries such as stress fractures and overuse syndromes.
- Chronic muscle soreness, joint stiffness, and overall fatigue.
- The female athlete triad symptoms.

Note: This list is certainly not designed to diagnose exercise addiction. Nearly everyone who trains regularly has experienced some of these symptoms at one time or another. However, their presence may serve as a warning and should not be ignored.

altogether). This might sound like a delightful prospect, but it is not something to aspire to. Without the periodic shedding of its glandular lining, the uterus becomes abnormally thickened, a condition known as uterine hyperplasia. Uterine hyperplasia can lead to serious health risks, including uterine cancer. Women who experience amenorrhea as a result of overtraining are often advised to undergo progesterone administration three or four times a year to induce a period or withdrawal cycle. Periodic menses, even if medically induced, will help prevent the development of uterine hyperplasia. If you are not pregnant and have missed three or more consecutive periods, you should seek medical attention.

How Can You Avoid Addiction?

To avoid developing compulsive habits, emphasize quality and intensity in your training rather than quantity and duration. Take off at least one day per week for rest. Do not curtail your caloric intake on rest days. Your muscles use the time off to resupply glycogen stores with the carbohydrates you would normally burn during your workout. For every gram of retained glycogen, three grams of water will also be recruited. However, any increase in body weight on your day off reflects better-fueled muscles, not fat gain.

A rigid training schedule is neither a substitute for nor tantamount to a rich and satisfying life. The healthy, well-balanced individual enjoys career, hobbies, friends, relationships, intellectual pursuits, and physical activity. Compulsive exercising can push all other aspects of life to the barely discernible periphery, until existence becomes a dark, endless tunnel of oppressive activity. If you are concerned about your eating or exercise habits, I urge you to seek help by consulting your health care provider.

TAKE IT OUTSIDE!

In Chapter 7, I briefly explained how I managed to transform from a very muscular 145-pound bodybuilder to a lean, toned 130-pound spokesmodel in a matter of months. My method entailed lots of cross-training and virtually no strength training for almost a year. I mentioned that I'd made a decision (to retire from bodybuilding), which led to a discovery (I'd spent years overtraining) that resulted in a revelation: Contrary to conventional wisdom, you can actually

SELF-ASSESSMENT QUIZ
How Healthy Are Your Exercise Habits?

Select the response that most accurately describes your relationship with exercise. Be honest in your self assessment.

1. How much time do you spend training in a day?

	POINTS
A. Less than 30 minutes	0
B. 30 minutes to 1 hour	1
C. 1 to 2 hours	2
D. Over 2 hours	3

2. How many times per week do you train?

	POINTS
A. Less than 3	0
B. 3 or 4	1
C. 5 or 6	2
D. Every day	3

3. How do you rate exercise as a priority in your life?

	POINTS
A. Less important than most other aspects of my life	0
B. Less important than work and relationships	1
C. Equally as important as work and relationships	2
D. It is the biggest priority in my life.	3

4. Why do you exercise?

	POINTS
A. Primarily for enjoyment	0
B. For health and enjoyment	1
C. For health; I don't really enjoy training	2
D. For the feeling of control it gives me	3

5. What would compel you to miss a workout?

	POINTS
A. I need a compelling reason to catch a workout	0
B. Injury, sickness, fatigue, work, social events	1
C. Injury or work only	2
D. Nothing short of death	3

6. If I overeat, I

	POINTS
A. Take it easy; who wants to train on a full stomach!	0
B. Exercise like usual	1
C. Do a little extra cardio	2
D. Exercise to burn off at least as many calories as I gained	3

7. When I miss a workout, I

	POINTS
A. Don't really care	0
B. Make a special effort not to miss the next one	1
C. Make it up	2
D. Rabid wolves couldn't keep me from a workout!	3

8. Family, friends, and coworkers

	POINTS
A. Don't even know that I work out	0
B. Are aware that I work out	1
C. Compliment me on my dedication to working out	2
D. Say that I have lost perspective and work out to excess	3

9. I generally date people

	POINTS
A. Whether they exercise or not	0
B. Who exercise a couple times a week to stay fit	1
C. Who find working out as important as I do	2
D. Who treat exercise as a way of life	3

10. My periods are

	POINTS
A. As predictable as Old Faithful	0
B. Fairly regular	1
C. Irregular	2
D. Periods? Haven't had one in months	3

Scoring

Add up the total number of points your answers have given you, and compare to the listings on the following page.

Below 7 points:
You have little to worry about in the way of exercise addiction. If you decide to up the intensity of your training routine, do it gradually to avoid injury.

7 to 15 points:
You likely enjoy a balanced approach to fitness with a healthy dedication to exercise. Keep up the good work.

16 to 20 points:
You are hard core and committed when it comes to your workouts, and you probably have some compulsive tendencies. If you begin to sense that "the tail is wagging the dog," it's time to reassess your priorities. Remember, exercise is supposed to make you feel healthy and invigorated, not anxious and enslaved. Also, be careful to avoid overtraining. If you find you are losing enthusiasm for your workouts or if you are constantly tired or sore, it's time for a break.

Over 20 points:
This quiz is by no means designed to make a medical diagnosis. However, your responses indicate that you exhibit potentially unhealthy training patterns. Please consider consulting a competent health professional.

stay in great shape without spending much time in a gym. In fact, you can do it the same way you did as a kid, simply by *playing*!

Over the years, I've determined that I am truly happiest when left to my own devices. I've never been able to hold a 9-to-5 job without tearing my hair out. I function poorly on teams. The only thing I find more distasteful than giving orders is following them. I have an overwhelming need to manage my own time. This has probably been the single greatest driving force, as well as the single largest obstacle, of my existence. It's why I became a writer. It has a lot to do with the fact that I am still single. (People like me aren't known for their diplomacy or their ability to compromise.) I don't have, nor do I particularly desire, any offspring. As a result, compared to just about every other woman I know, my schedule is marvelously free and flexible.

In terms of deadlines and other work responsibilities, I am reliable, punctual, and consistent in my efforts to do the best possible job. By the same token, the only time clock I punch is internal. Having the latitude to set my own hours is crucial to my performance because I am infinitely more creative, focused, and productive between sundown and sunup than at any other time of day. When I finally tumble into bed during the wee hours of the morning, it is with the delicious knowledge that my phone is unplugged and the alarm is not set. Obviously, not everyone has such luxury.

But even in my carefully constructed Peter Pan world, the demands of career, friends, and family occasionally preclude spending an entire afternoon on a bike ride. The gym is without a doubt the most time-efficient means to simultaneously improve muscle tone and cardiovascular health. However, I firmly believe that everyone can benefit from the wonders of outdoor activity. Especially if you happen to be one of the thousands who carry a self-imposed prison sentence to the gym with them day after monotonous day. I don't care how much interesting equipment your prison possesses. If barbells and treadmills are your only form of exercise, traipsing to the gym day in and day out eventually becomes bland and tiresome.

I urge even the busiest person to make an effort to reclaim at least one day a week to devote to outdoor enjoyment. Which, by the way, brings me to that life-altering epiphany I alluded to earlier. If you'll indulge me for a moment while I wax philosophical . . . By nature, I am restless, driven, and neurotic. It's often difficult for me to put stress out of my mind and simply enjoy the process of life. Sports are one of the few things that keep me firmly anchored in the moment. When I'm sailing through the air on a snowboard, dropping down a rock ledge on my mountain bike, or being battered by a ten-foot wave, I'm not thinking about deadlines, the fight I had with my boyfriend, or the million bucks I have yet to earn. It's all about the moment. Find it. Then live it!

The following are brief descriptions of my all-time favorite outdoor activities and their physique-enhancing powers. The estimated caloric expenditures indicated below each activity are based on a 150-pound individual.

• ROLLER BLADING •

What you need to get started: blades

Also recommended: knee pads, elbow pads, wrist guards, bike or skate helmet

Why it's fun: Roller blading is an enormously cardiovascular activity that requires a minimum investment of time to become relatively proficient. It affords you the opportunity to get out and see the sights while you tone your lower body.

Physique benefits: Build that backside! The gluteal complex is actually a combination of three distinct muscles: the gluteus maximus, gluteus minimus, and gluteus medius. The gluteus medius and minimus are hip abductors (used to extend the legs laterally out to the side). They are called upon when the leg is lifted to the side, as in a push off during skating.

Estimated caloric expenditure: 350 to 400 calories per hour (at 9 mph; once you have the hang of it, you'll go a lot faster and burn even more calories!)

• ROLLER/ICE HOCKEY •

What you need to get started: skates or blades, knee/shin pads, hockey gloves, hockey helmet, stick, puck or ball

Also recommended: elbow pads, chest protection, padded shorts, mouth guard

Why it's fun: Once you've mastered the basics of skating, nothing improves your skills faster than playing hockey. Stick handling is another story! It could take a while before you feel confident playing against opponents. I find the best way to practice is to get two or three friends together and find a parking lot.

Physique benefits: As with roller blading, hockey targets the glutes, especially the gluteus medius and minimus. The crouched position, side-to-side motion, and stick handling will also work your quads, shoulders, low back, and abdominal muscles.

Estimated caloric expenditure: 800 to 1,000 calories per hour (if you don't take any breaks)

SKIING

What you need to get started: skis, boots, bindings, poles, winter wear

Why it's fun: Speed, speed, and more speed! When the hill is too icy for snowboarding, I grab the skis and just *go* . . . like a bat out of hell!

Physique benefits: Quads, get ready for the biggest challenge you've ever faced. Glutes and hams, you'll feel it too!

Estimated caloric expenditure: 300 to 400 calories per hour (stopping for beers at the lodge doesn't count)

SNOWBOARDING

What you need to get started: snowboard, boots, bindings, winter wear

Why it's fun: I have never in my entire life gotten more of a rush from any activity than I've gotten from snowboarding. For all its complexity (and the better you get, the more there is to learn), the fundamentals of snowboarding can be mastered in a matter of days. Unlike skiing, the initial learning curve is steep. So unless you're an Olympic level skier, chances are excellent that you will be a better snowboarder than you ever were a skier by the end of your first season.

Physique benefits: If looking and feeling fit is your top priority, snowboarding will whittle your glutes, build your calves, and chisel definition into your quads and hams like nobody's business.

Estimated caloric expenditure: 300 to 400 calories per hour

MOUNTAIN BIKING

What you need to get started: mountain bike, bike helmet, gloves, patch kit, hydration system

Recommended for extreme riding: full-face helmet, body armor, mouth guard, eye protection

Why it's fun: Remember what I said about the unbeatable rush I get from snowboarding? I lied. Downhill mountain biking gives me just as big of a rush. Technical trail riding is the most cranial sport I've ever tried. Depending on the degree of difficulty of the terrain, mountain biking can be anything from a simple ride in the park to a death-defying adventure as you hurtle over rock faces, clear log piles, and follow narrow planks high into the branches of trees. Regardless of how extreme you plan to go, mountain biking is a fast-paced workout that the whole family can enjoy.

Physique benefits: Your butt, calves, and quads will never look better. If you take it extreme, your shoulders, triceps, and lats will get a workout as well.

Estimated caloric expenditure: 600 to 700 calories per hour

• MOUNTAIN HIKING •

What you need to get started: all-terrain footwear, comfortable clothing

Also recommended: bug spray, hydration system, bear bells in bear country

Why it's fun: As far as alpine sports go, hiking may not be as exciting as mountain biking or snowboarding, but it sure is a great way to spend a lazy summer day. Imagine enjoying hours of breathtaking sights as you climb to the summit. You're guaranteed to return to sea level feeling refreshed and relaxed. Pack a camera, food, warm clothing, your best friend/boyfriend/dog, and make a day of it.

Physique benefits: Walking uphill works your quads, calves, and glutes in a way that resistance training cannot. If you don't believe me, notice how sore you are the day after a long hike.

Estimated caloric expenditure: 400 calories per hour (for sustained hiking in uphill terrain)

• CROSS-COUNTRY SKIING •

What you need to get started: cross-country skis, poles, boots, bindings, winter wear

Why it's fun: I first tried cross-country skiing after an ankle injury prevented me from snowboarding for a few weeks. Imagine my surprise when my "rehab" turned out to be a total blast! As a rule, people who like to run love to cross-country ski. Me, I'm not a huge fan of running, and I didn't expect to be terribly intrigued by cross-country skiing. I was delightfully mistaken. It's fast paced, cardiovascularly demanding, and kind to the joints. Even though I'm appallingly bad at it, it's still my single most favorite thing to do in a snowy forest under a starlit sky. Bring your friends and hit the hot tub afterward. You'll be glad you did.

Physique benefits: Cross-country skiing places enormous demands on your butt, shoulders, and anterior tibialis (the tear-shaped muscle that lies over your shin) as well as your lungs.

Estimated caloric expenditure: 600 to 700 calories per hour

SURFING

What you need to get started: surf board, leash, rugged swim wear

Also recommended for cooler climates: wet suit, booties

Why it's fun: How can it not be? The outfits are sensational (who doesn't love surf shorts?) and you get to ogle loads of scantily clad guys while they show off for you. As for other amusing sea creatures, I've sighted sea lions, dolphins, and, once a whale, all while surfing the shores of Los Angeles County. Not to mention that absolute exhilaration you feel when you actually manage to catch and ride a wave.

Physique benefits: The two Ls: lungs and lats. Paddling through the ocean while being pummeled by waves is one of the more physically demanding things I've ever attempted. I am a horrendous surfer and I get an amazing workout just trying to swim out to the line up. I go for (and miss) lots of waves to ensure that I never stop paddling.

Estimated caloric expenditure: 500 calories per hour (for sustained paddling)

One Addict's Story of Triumph
(as told to Christine Lydon, M.D.)

This is the true account of a woman I interviewed in 1999 while research-
ing an article on the topic of exercise addiction. Unfortunately, her story is
far from unique. Fortunately, in her case at least, it has a happy ending.

I guess it all started about the time I finished college and joined the workforce. In school, I had a really healthy attitude about exercise. I played
coed basketball and softball, more because they were a blast than as a
means to stay in shape. I also lifted weights on and off because I liked the
way strength training shaped my narrow shoulders and toned my thighs.
It never made me feel guilty to miss a workout or a game because I had
to study for an exam, or I was tired, or I had a date. I was fit and healthy
and I looked it. I didn't spend much time obsessing about my body.

After I graduated, everything changed. The carefree, flexible life I'd
enjoyed as a student was gone forever. I got a very time-consuming job
working for a software company, and my career became my central focus.
It seemed like I never had time to play sports or have fun anymore. After
about six months, I had gained 20 pounds and grown disgusted with my
body. I also felt like my life wasn't mine anymore. My solution? I joined a
gym and threw myself into weight training.

At first it was great. My time off had really primed my body and my
muscles grew like gangbusters. After a few months, I decided to take my
training up a notch and do something about the flab on my stomach and
thighs. That's when I discovered "cardio." What a concept: Climb onto a
machine that is going nowhere and run like a crazed hamster. I started
with half an hour three times a week and the weight came off. I liked the
changes in my body and was disappointed when my weight eventually
plateaud. I knew I'd have to up my intensity to keep getting leaner, so I
started doing cardio every day. Then I increased the duration of my sessions until I was climbing imaginary stairs or rowing an imaginary boat for
at least an hour and a half every Monday through Sunday. And when it
came to throwing around the iron, I would sooner eat worms than miss
my daily lifting fix. I was tired and sore a lot, but I preferred to feel sore
than to feeling guilty that I might not have trained hard enough.

My exercising soon began to invade other aspects of my life. I would not go out with a guy who didn't train because I figured if I worked this hard to be attractive and sexy, he better be doing the same. Most of my relationships were short-lived. The guys who I deemed adequate physical specimens were always so obsessed with training that we could never find time to do much together besides work out. And beyond training, we didn't seem to have much to talk about. There was a time when I loved to read, but I got to a point where my only forms of literature were fitness and muscle magazines. I couldn't recall the last time I'd actually finished a book. I wouldn't accept invitations to dinner because I was afraid the restaurant wouldn't have "clean" alternatives. I was reluctant to make social plans in case I might need the time to fit in a workout. I was completely spent by the time I fell into bed at night, and the first thing I did in the morning was run to the mirror to see if the definition in my quads was any more noticeable. It's disturbing for me to look back at my outlandish behavior and realize that I got nothing but positive reinforcement from the people around me. Everyone complimented my dedication and said how they wished they had the discipline to work out as much as me. My social circle gradually shrank until it included only those people I knew from the gym.

On the outside, I guess everything appeared relatively normal. I was excelling at my job; my body looked great; and I carried myself with a facade of confidence. On the inside, I was wretchedly unhappy. I hated my job and my manipulative, controlling boss. My muscles were sore every minute of the day. My caloric intake was far below what my activity level demanded, yet I was having an increasingly difficult time staying lean. I was terrified that I would never achieve the perfect physique, that I would get fat and ugly the minute I stopped training to exhaustion. My mood was labile; one minute angry, then depressed, then anxious. I was lonely and miserable and didn't know where to turn.

To this day, I'm not sure what finally sparked me to take my body back. I guess it started when I quit my job in favor of freelance work. I was financially strapped at first and decided not to renew my gym membership when it expired. Instead, I dusted off my bike and started using it as an alternative form of exercise. I joined a softball team. I learned how to ski. I remembered what it felt like to *love* exercise. My "recovery" didn't happen overnight, and there were many moments of trepidation along the way. Sometimes I would be so riddled with guilt after skipping work outs for two or three days in a row that I would drive to the local high school and run laps around the track in the middle of the night.

Today, I feel I have regained a healthy perspective. I bike just about everywhere. I play on two softball teams and play pickup basketball a couple times a week. I engage in light to moderate strength training at my home gym two or three times a week. I no longer feel anxiety if work or some other obligation keeps me inactive for a couple days. If I'm sick, or tired, or injured, I don't train. I am in better shape, both physically and emotionally, than I have ever been in my life. I still eat clean, but I no longer torment myself about every gram of fat or crumb of bread that passes my lips. In fact, I'm actually leaner now than I was at the height of my infatuation with the Stair Master. I have rediscovered my love for reading, sketching, and watching old movies. I'm aware that I have a compulsive personality and that I need to be wary of falling into unhealthy habits. But more than that, I know I have the strength to face my demons and win. I wouldn't go back to the way things were for all the quad definition in the world!

PART III

The Movements

A Bodacious Back
and Beautiful Biceps

Back training is one of the most underrated means for developing a sensational physique. A V-shaped back not only accentuates a small waist, it can also make a thick waist appear thinner. Moreover, back training is one of the most effective ways to building good posture. The tensile forces exerted by toned back muscles tend to pull the scapulae back, eradicating the droopy shouldered, hunched look to which so many modern women succumb. In a word, back training can undo much of the damage caused by a desk job. Back training targets literally dozens of muscles, from those responsible for keeping your spine properly aligned to those empowering you with the ability to pull objects to you. However, for the purposes of describing strength training for the back, I will limit my discussion to two main muscle groups: the latissimus dorsi and the spinal erectors.

Taken as a single muscle group, the back boasts an intricate multitude of interlocking, overlapping layers. But for all its complexity, the back is surprisingly impotent without the biceps. Just as each limb is, in many ways, merely a functional extension of the torso, the biceps are, in many ways, merely functional extensions of the back muscles. When we use our back muscles, our biceps usually contribute to the effort. Consider, for example, rowing a boat, reigning in a poorly trained rottweiler, or playing tug-o-war. Our spinal erectors contract to stabilize our torso, our latissimus muscles resists the opposing drag, and the biceps contract, resulting in elbow flexion, which pulls the opposing force closer to our center of gravity. This amplifies our control over the opposing force and increases the efficiency of our energy expenditure.

FUNCTIONAL ANATOMY OF THE BACK AND BICEPS

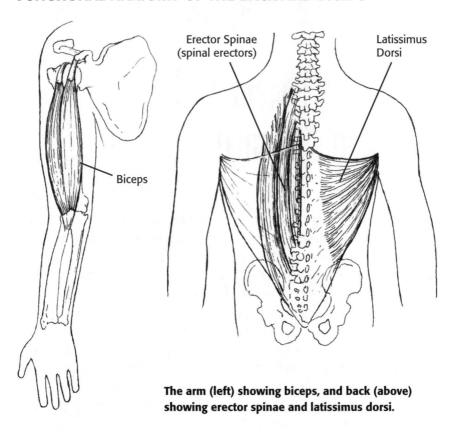

The arm (left) showing biceps, and back (above) showing erector spinae and latissimus dorsi.

Spinal Erectors

The erector spinae muscles, or spinal erectors, are the extensor muscles of the spine. They run longitudinally, interconnecting bones of the spine, ribs, skull, and pelvis. The spinal erectors stabilize your spine. Most movements targeting these muscles involve spinal extension, such as when you arch your back. Typically, resistance exercises that call most heavily on the spinal erectors also involve the latissimus muscles.

Latissimus Dorsi

The latissimus dorsi is a large, flat muscle that attaches the back of the trunk to the humerus (upper arm bone). It originates on the lower thoracic vertebrae and pelvis and wraps around the upper arm, inserting onto the anterior (front) aspect of the top of the humerus. Its actions include humerus adduction (bringing the upper arm against the trunk) and medial rotation of the humerus (rotating the upper arm inward). Working in conjunction with the pectoral muscles, the latissimus muscles bring the trunk toward the arms, as when performing a chin-up.

Biceps Brachii

The biceps brachii muscle is one of the most responsive muscle groups in the body; even beginners will have little trouble isolating it. The biceps brachii muscle has two heads, hence the appellation *bi-ceps.* One head lies on top of the other and, when flexed, lends the upper arm its ball-shaped peak. Because of the way the biceps insert onto the radial bone of the lower arm, the biceps not only flex the arm at the elbow but also supinate (pronounced *soup-innate*) the forearm. To illustrate suppination, hold your arm straight out, with

A Brief Lesson in Muscle Anatomy

Muscle is made up of thousands of longitudinal fibers. The middle portion of the muscle, or the muscle belly, is the thickest part of the muscle because it contains the greatest number of muscle fibers. Many muscles consist of two or more distinct sections, each referred to as a separate head. At both ends of every head, muscle tissue blends with connective tissue to form tendons. Tendons, in turn, attach to bones. When a muscle contracts, the muscle belly shortens and becomes thicker, exerting forces (via the tendons) that bring the different bones closer together.

For a given muscle, the bony attachment closest to the midline of the torso comprises the muscle's proximal attachment, sometimes referred to as the muscle's origin. The bony attachment farthest from the midline of the torso comprises the muscle's distal attachment or insertion. For example, the origin or proximal attachment of the long head of the biceps muscle is the humerus (the upper arm bone), and the insertion or distal attachment of the long head of the biceps is the radius (the bone on the thumb side of the lower arm).

your palm facing down. Now, without flexing your elbow, turn your hand so that your palm faces up, as if you were holding a bowl of soup. You have just suppinated your forearm. If you pay close attention, you will notice that your biceps flex slightly even though your elbow doesn't bend. In order to work the full range of motion of the biceps, you must both flex your elbow and suppinate your forearm. It's not absolutely necessary to accomplish this with every single exercise, but I recommend incorporating at least one such movement each time you train biceps.

SYNERGISTIC MULTIJOINT POWER MOVEMENTS

Because all multijoint back exercises also tax the biceps, by starting with back, you begin to fatigue your biceps even before you target them. Hence, by training these synergistic groups during the same session, you increase your efficiency, and the number of single-joint power movements necessary to fatigue your biceps falls with each back-targeting multijoint power movement. Essentially, when you train back with 6 to 8 sets of multijoint power movements, you are also doing the equivalent of 3 to 4 sets of power movements for your biceps. The split routines listed in Appendix C are structured to take this overlap into account.

Lat Cable Pull-Down

One of the most common exercises for back development is the lat cable pull-down, so called because it targets the latissimus dorsi, better known as "lats" in gym vernacular. There are at least a dozen ways to do lat cable pull downs. However, if your goal is back development, only a few of these methods support your objectives. Like chin-ups, pull-downs are a composite, multijoint exercise that calls on lats, pecs, biceps, and forearms. Many people train their back ineffectively, and pull-downs are a major culprit. The straighter you sit, the more you rely on your chest and trapezius (upper back) muscles. Instead, you should lean back slightly. If you use a reverse grip, with your palms facing you, you are placing your biceps at a mechanical advantage. Instead, to maximize the latissimus contribution, grip the bar with your palms facing away and your hands spaced widely apart. Use a weight that permits perfect form.

Your spine should remain relatively stationary during the exer-

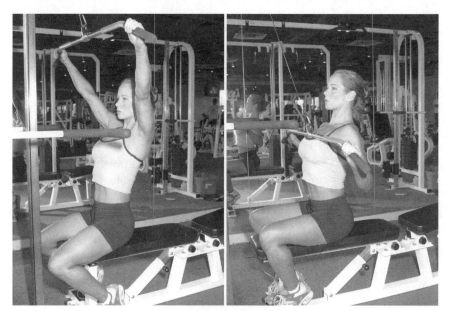

Lat-Cable Pulldown

cise. Resist the temptation to rock back and forth as you move from the eccentric (pulling the weight down) to the concentric (letting the weight rise) phase of the motion. Unlike most other exercises, you should inhale during the concentric phase, as you pull the bar to your upper chest for an isometric (muscular tension without further movement) half count. Control the weight during the eccentric phase; don't let the cable pull you upright. As always, concentrate on isolating your lats and feeling them work.

You may notice that your biceps and pectorals are called into play during the pull-down. Latissimus training inevitably involves auxiliary muscle groups. In order to maximize latissimus contribution, I recommend that you treat each latissimus exercise as if it were a defining or finishing exercise and stay within a higher rep range. Refrain from concentrating on these auxiliary muscle groups. When you are targeting lats, create a strong mind-body connection specifically with your lats.

Pull-downs to the rear of the neck place the glenohumeral (shoulder) joint in an unnatural degree of external rotation and can lead to strains, rotator cuff injury, and eventually, arthritis. I recommend avoiding them altogether.

🏠 Wide-Grip Chin-Ups

Wide grip chin-ups are a more advanced movement used to target the lats. As with pull-downs, use a wide, palms-out grip and pull yourself up to the point where your upper chest contacts the bar.

When first attempting this rather difficult movement, it's helpful to have a training partner available to lift you from the ankles should you "stall out" mid-rep. Your partner should provide you with only just enough help to complete each individual repetition. Use your own strength for the eccentric phase as you slowly lower yourself back to the starting position.

If you don't have a training partner, you can "spot" yourself by bending your knees and resting your toes on a chair placed behind you. As you pull yourself up to the bar, extend your legs and use your toes to provide assistance.

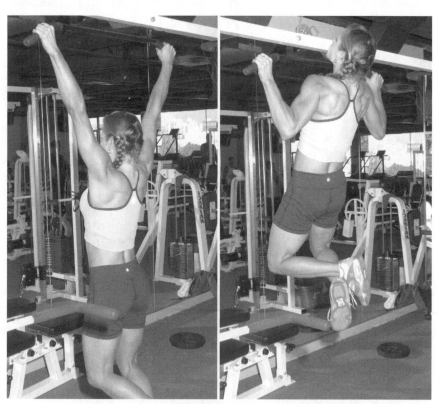

Wide-Grip Chin-ups

 This icon indicates home-friendly exercises.

T-Bar Rows

Unlike pull-downs and chin-ups, with T-bar rows your chest is anchored firmly (against the machine), making it a little more difficult to cheat with momentum. I recommend a wide overhand grip to minimize the biceps' contribution. At the start of the movement, hold your head and neck steady, stick out your chest, and keep your shoulders back. Inhale as you pull the weight evenly toward your chest. Pause for an isometric count at the peak of the excursion before exhaling and slowly returning to the starting position. As always, concentrate on feeling the exercise in your lats.

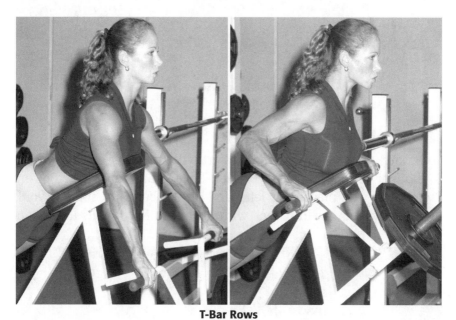

T-Bar Rows

🏠 Bent-Over Barbell Rows

Start with the empty bar to get a feel for the motion before adding any weight. Firmly plant your feet approximately shoulders-width apart. Bend at the knees to lift the bar with a wide, overhand grip. Keeping your knees slightly bent, bend at the waist so that your torso forms a 90° angle with your thighs. Keeping your back straight, head up, and elbows out, lift the barbell until it contacts your torso. Pause for a brief isometric count, then lower the bar to the starting position.

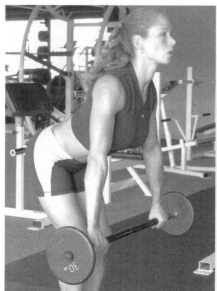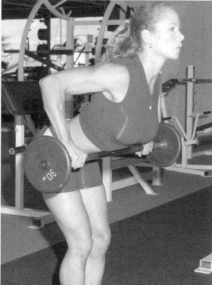

Bent-Over Barbell Rows

⌂ Bent-Over Dumbbell Rows

To properly execute this exercise, start with a low, flat bench. Kneel to the rear of the bench on your left knee. Plant your right foot on the ground, and place your left hand on the bench to support your upper body. Grip the dumbbell with your right hand while it rests on

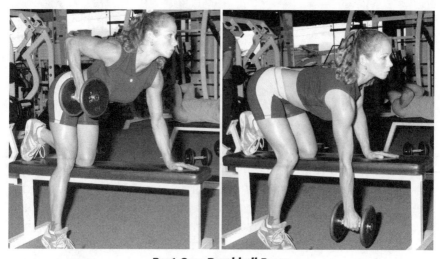

Bent-Over Dumbbell Rows

the floor. You will have to reach for it, letting your shoulder drop as your arm extends. From this starting position, keep your right arm at your side as you flex your elbow, raise your shoulder, and twist your spine slightly, bringing the weight up until it is parallel to your torso. (As with other back exercises, remember to inhale, not exhale, during the concentric phase.) At this point of full contraction, your elbow should actually be pointing above your torso. (It might help to think of this movement as similar to pulling the start-up cord on a lawn mower.) Give a full two-count isometric squeeze at the peak of the motion. Exhale as you lower the weight slowly and steadily to a point just short of where it would make contact with the floor. Repeat to fatigue, then switch sides.

You will feel this exercise in your biceps, lats, and middle back (spinal erectors). Concentrate on your lats and middle back, especially during the isometric contraction at the top of the motion.

Cable Rows

Cable rows are my all-time personal favorite back exercise. At the start of the movement, your arms should be fully extended, your back flexed forward, your hips and feet firmly planted on the padded seat and foot stage, respectively. Inhale as you straighten your spine, extending it against the weight of the machine. As your spine arcs back, stick your chest out and pull the weight toward your abdomen. Keep your shoulders down and back straight to prevent cheating with your trapezius muscles. Concentrate on feeling the power coming from your lats, not your arm, chest, or neck muscles. Hold the

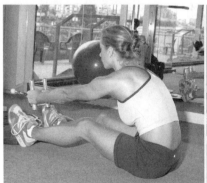
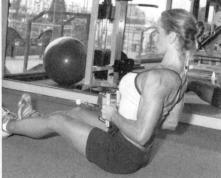

Cable Rows

weight for an isometric count at the peak of the excursion. Exhale as you slowly and steadily return to your starting position.

REVIEW Tips for Building a Bodacious Back

1. For pull-downs, chin-ups, and T-bar rows, use a wide, palms-out grip on the bar.

2. When training the lats, concentrate on feeling the contraction in your lats, not your chest, biceps, or trapezius muscles.

3. Don't let the weight spring back during the eccentric phase of your back exercises. Control it with a slow, steady release of the contraction.

4. For back exercises, utilize the opposite of your normal breathing pattern: Inhale during the concentric phase and exhale during the eccentric phase.

BICEPS POWER MOVEMENTS

Women used to go out of their way to deliver the following back-handed compliment to those of us with muscular arms: "Your arms look great. I don't train mine because I'm afraid they'd get too big." Then a funny thing happened. *Terminator 2* and a sculpted Linda Hamilton exploded onto the big screen. Suddenly these same women were flocking to me for advice. "Your arms look great!" they'd declare. "How can I get mine bigger?" We who sported a pair of loaded guns before Linda Hamilton made it trendy could have told you all a long time ago that the vast majority of the opposite sex (men and women alike) find muscular, defined arms extremely sexy. Arms are, without a doubt, the body part I enjoy training the most. Following is a list of my favorite arm exercises. Try them, and enjoy the results.

🏠 Alternating Dumbbell Curls

Alternating dumbbell curls can be done standing or seated. If you perform them while standing, be sure to bend your knees slightly and pay strict attention to form or you'll be asking for a back injury. If you prefer to do this exercise while seated, I recommend using a bench with the back at a slight incline. By leaning back, sticking out

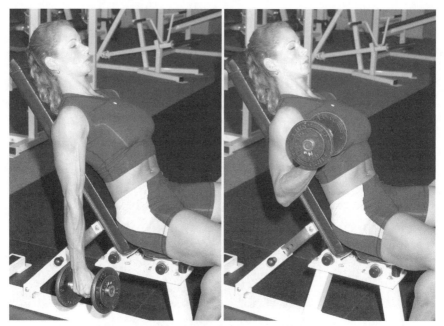

Alternating Dumbbell Curls (Seated)

your chest, and keeping your elbows tightly at your sides, it becomes nearly impossible to injure yourself or cheat with trapezius muscles or lats.

Standing or seated, bring the dumbbells up one at a time. Control the weights; never jerk or swing them. Momentum does not build muscle, but it does injure joints. Exhale as you contract your biceps. Squeeze your biceps for an isometric half-count at the top of the motion. Inhale as you lower the dumbbell to the start position.

By varying your grip slightly, it's possible to tax all the different fibers of your biceps. With the conventional grip, you start with the dumbbells lowered and your palms facing your sides. As you raise each dumbbell, twist your arm so that, at the top of the motion, your palm is facing the front of your chest. In other words, supinate your forearm while flexing your elbow. The hammer grip, which looks just like it sounds, does not incorporate supination, so that at the top of the motion your palms are still facing your sides.

🏠 Barbell Curls

Barbell curls are best performed standing. As with alternating curls,

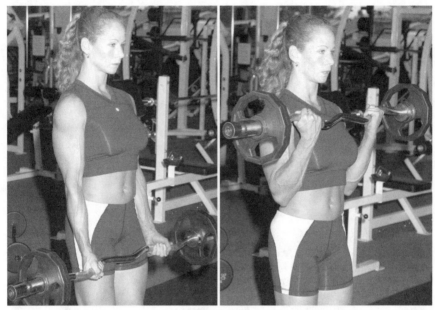

Barbell Curls

bend your knees slightly, keep your chest out, shoulders back, and pay strict attention to form to avoid back strain and cheating. Don't rock your body to raise the bar; all the power should come from your biceps. Because it puts less strain on your wrists, I recommend using an e-z bar rather than a straight bar.

Preacher Curls

Because the very nature of the apparatus discourages cheating, preacher curls are highly effective at emphasizing the biceps' insertion onto the radius. To avoid straining your biceps, use a weight that allows you to accomplish the movement from the fully extended position. For added pump, give an isometric squeeze at the top of the movement before commencing the eccentric phase of the contraction.

BICEPS DEFINING MOVEMENTS: PIQUE THE PEAK

The exercises found in this section include those movements that are most effective at building the biceps' "peak." Unlike dumbbell or barbell curls, where you experience maximum resistance prior to maximum muscular contraction, these exercises require the greatest

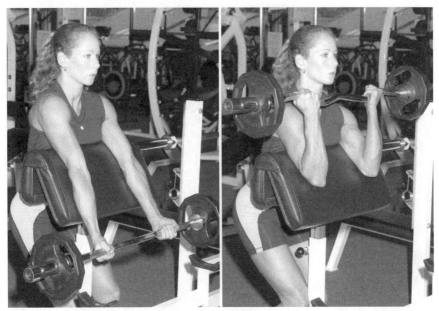

Preacher Curls

effort at the top of the movement. For this reason, they are extremely useful for adding height to the biceps and bestowing a toned, round, shape.

🏠 Concentration Curls

Start by leaning forward and bracing your elbow against the inside of your knee. Your arm should be fully extended at the start position. Now simply curl the dumbbell up toward your shoulder. Hold it for a half-count at the top and squeeze. Use a relatively light weight to prevent cheating with momentum.

Overhead Cable Curls

Using cables, you will experience similar resistance throughout the length of the excursion. Overhead cable curls are a great finishing exercise and should be done with a relatively light weight. This exercise requires a bilateral cable apparatus with stirrup attachments (see high-to-low cable flyes page 197). If the cable pulleys are adjustable, set both sides for maximum height. To begin, hold one stirrup in each hand, position yourself at the midline of the apparatus, and fully extend your arms above your shoulders to form a skyward

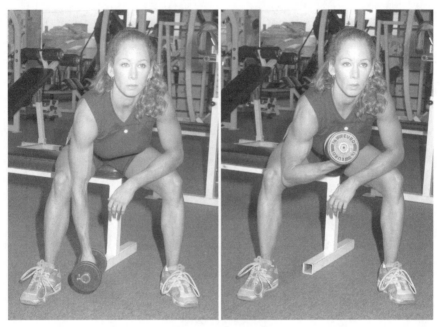

Concentration Curls

V shape. If you are too tall to acheive an adequate V with your arms (that is, your V looks more like a horizontal line), sink to a kneeling position. Then, using a palms up grip, flex your biceps against the resistance and curl the stirrups toward your ears. Throughout the excursion, your humeri (upper arms) should remain stationary relative to your scapulae (shoulders) and should neither sink nor rise. Likewise, your elbows should never move forward relative to your torso. If you can see your elbows in the periphery of your visual range without turning your head, they are too far forward and you are cheating with pectoral muscles. To minimize pectoral involvement, stand forward relative to the plane of the machine. This moves the force vector behind your head, making it more difficult for your elbows to collapse inward.

REVIEW Tips for Building Beautiful Biceps

1. In order to work the full range of motion of the biceps, you must both flex your elbow and supinate your forearm. Incorporate at least one such movement each time you train biceps.

2. When performing barbell or alternating curls, keep your back straight, stick your chest out, and hold your elbows tightly at your sides to avoid injury and cheating with trapezius and latissimus muscles.

3. For defining the peak of the biceps, try exercises that offer maximum resistance at the top of the motion.

Pump Up Your Posture

Slouching and poor posture can stretch spinal ligaments and shorten the chest muscles, exaggerating the natural concave curve of the thoracic (middle) spine. This condition, known as postural kyphosis, is often accompanied by "swayback," or hyperlordosis, of the lumbar (lower) spine as it compensates by curving excessively in the opposite direction. Postural kyphosis is very common among sedentary young women. Ignored, it can lead to serious health issues, including back pain, decreased lung capacity, and, in severe cases, neurological symptoms.

Postural kyphosis can be prevented and even reversed by practicing healthy body mechanics to correct posture:

• When seated in a chair, your knees should be level with or slightly above your hips, with your feet flat on the floor.

• Computer screens and reading materials should be at eye level to help keep your back straight and your head high.

• When driving, sit firmly against the seat back and adjust the head rest so that it supports the middle of your head.

• When standing in one place or waiting in line, frequently shift your weight from one foot to the other. If possible, place one foot on a raised platform, changing feet often. Do not lock your knees.

• Always walk with your shoulders back, chest out, and head held high. Bend at the knees, not at the back, to lift heavy objects.

• When carrying a heavy object, hold it close to you.

- Frequently switch arms when using a shoulder bag.

- When sleeping on your back, place a pillow under your head and shoulders and a pillow under your knees. When sleeping on your side, place a pillow under your head so that your head is level with the rest of your spine. Also, place a pillow between your knees and keep them bent. Avoid sleeping on your stomach.

Regular exercise and daily stretching are the cornerstones to good posture. Exercises to strengthen the abdominal muscles and stretch the hamstrings are especially important to correct postural kyphosis. Basic crunches, which target the entire rectus abdominus, are the mainstay of abdominal development. See Chapter 11 for instruction.

To stretch your hamstrings, stand with your legs about shoulder width apart. Keeping your knees slightly bent, bend forward at the hips, letting your neck and arms relax. Descend until you feel a stretch in your hamstrings. Do not go beyond the point of mild discomfort. Stretching should not be painful! Hold the stretch for 20 seconds, then slowly ascend to the starting position. Keeping your heels flat, feet parallel, and head high, bend your knees until you feel your quads engage. Hold the standing bent-knee position for 20 seconds. Repeat the entire process for at least 10 reps daily.

To improve overall muscle tone and strength, begin low-impact activities, such as swimming, cycling, and walking. Increase the intensity and duration of your workouts gradually to prevent injury. Any new or worsening symptoms of thoracic curvature warrant a visit to your health care provider.

Spectacular Pectorals, Shapely Shoulders, and Terrific Triceps

Training the pectoral muscles is every bit as important as training any other muscle group. While strength training will not increase breast tissue, it can enhance your breasts by building the muscle that lies underneath. Even if you are well endowed, poorly toned pectoral muscles can make your chest appear sunken. In addition, chest training is just about the best way to naturally enhance your cleavage line. Aesthetics aside, your pec muscles are utilized in virtually every upper body movement you perform in real life, from vacuuming to carrying heavy objects (kids, groceries, laundry), to pushing heavy objects (revolving doors, furniture, shopping carts), to playing sports like tennis, softball, and golf.

In much the same way that the latissimus muscles rely on the biceps, the pectoral muscles rely on the triceps and their ability to extend the elbow. The deltoid complex (shoulder muscles) also play a vital role in many "push" movements. When you push downward, as during a decline bench press, the primary movers are your pectoral muscles and triceps. On the other hand, when you push upward, as during a military press, the primary movers are your deltoid muscles and triceps. When you push straight forward, as during a flat bench press, you are exploiting both pectoral and deltoid input (not to mention the multitalented triceps). In a nutshell, there exists a gradual conversion from primarily pectoral input to primarily deltoid input as the vector of the "push" moves from below shoulder height to above shoulder height. The pecs and delts, as they're known familiarly, have an enormous overlap, and in virtually all cases are assisted by the triceps.

FUNCTIONAL ANATOMY OF THE CHEST, SHOULDERS, AND TRICEPS

The Pectoral Complex

The pectoral complex is composed of two separate muscles. The pectoral major is a large, triangular muscle that originates from the anterior (front) aspect of the clavicle (collarbone), sternum, and ribs and attaches to the upper part of the humerus (upper arm bone). Its actions include humeral adduction (bringing your arm to your side) and medial rotation of the humerus (turning your upper arm inward).

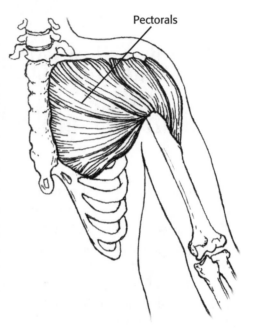

The chest showing pectorals.

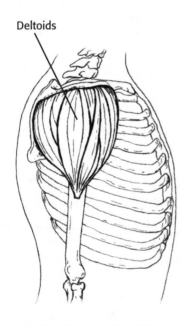

The shoulder showing deltoids.

The pectoral minor is a small, sail-shaped muscle that lies beneath the pectoral major. The fibers of the pectoral minor originate from ribs 3, 4, and 5 and attach to the scapular (shoulder blade). It acts primarily to draw the scapula forward against the chest wall.

The Deltoid Complex

The deltoid complex is a triangular muscle that originates from the spine of the scapula and the clavicle and inserts onto the upper portion of the humerus. The deltoid muscle is composed of three distinct heads:

the anterior head, the lateral head, and the posterior head. In a well-defined deltoid complex, the demarcation between the three divisions is obvious. The anterior head flexes and internally rotates the humerus relative to the shoulder (in other words, it raises your arm straight up in front of you). The lateral head is the largest of the three divisions. It abducts the humerus (that is, it raises your arm straight out to your side, like the wing of an airplane). The posterior head extends and laterally rotates the humerus (it brings your arm up and back, as if you were trying to bring your elbows together over your spine).

The Triceps

The triceps muscle has three heads. The medial (middle) head lies buried beneath the other two. The posterior head attaches to the scapula. It lies to the rear of its neighbors and makes up the bulk of the visible portion of the triceps, representing the back of the "horseshoe" shape of a well-defined triceps group. The anterior head forms the front of the horseshoe and inserts onto the humerus.

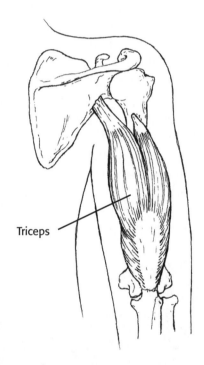

Triceps

The arm showing triceps.

The triceps function by extending the arm at the elbow and pronating the forearm. Pronation is the opposite of suppination and can be illustrated by holding your arm straight out in front of you, palm facing up. Place your opposite hand on your triceps as you flip your palm down. Although you have not extended your elbow, you should notice that your triceps contract slightly. (An interesting bit of trivia: Since the biceps are more powerful at suppination than the triceps are at pronation, a left-handed person will have more difficulty driving a screw, whereas a right-handed person will have more difficulty removing that screw.)

SYNERGISTIC MULTIJOINT POWER MOVEMENTS

Essentially, all multijoint power movements to target either the pectorals or the deltoids will also involve the triceps. When you train pecs or delts with 6 to 8 sets of multijoint power movements, you are also doing the equivalent of 3 or 4 sets of power movements for your triceps. The split routines listed in Appendix C are structured to take this overlap into account.

Incline, Decline, and Flat Dumbbell Press

Primary movers: **Pectorals**

I am always surprised by the number of people who lift weights and still consider the bench press to be the mainstay of chest training. For best results in terms of strength and development, it is important to duplicate the physiological range of motion. The bench press works only a narrow zone of pectoral range of motion, calling heavily on the anterior deltoid and triceps muscles. The natural, full range of motion of the pectoral complex brings your arm all the way across the midline of your body. If you hold your arm straight out to the side at shoulder height, invoking the pectoral muscles brings your hand across your body and past your opposite shoulder. With the bench press, the wide, locked grip of your hands on the bar prevents this movement. More-

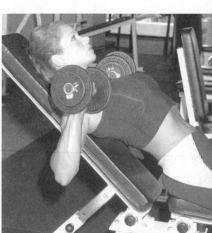
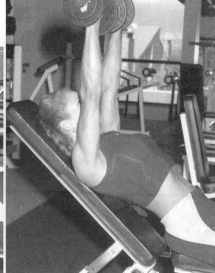

Incline Dumbbell Press

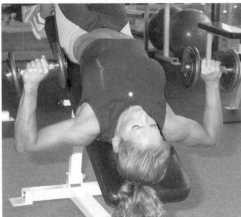

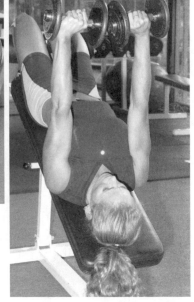

Decline Dumbbell Press

over, the stresses imposed by a rigid bar and heavy weight force your shoulder joint into an unnatural degree of external rotation as the bar is lowered onto the chest. This can be damaging to the tendons of the shallow glenohumeral (shoulder) joint, eventually leading to shoulder instability, injury, and arthritis.

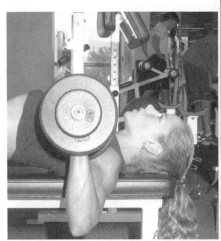

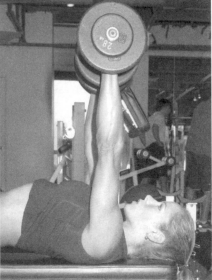

Flat Dumbbell Press

The best exercises for the pectoral complex permit your arms to approach one another at the midline at the peak of the excursion. I recommend incorporating primarily these movements into your routine, and starting your training with the most demanding movements. Free-weight exercises like the incline dumbbell press (torso elevated relative to legs), decline dumbbell press (legs elevated relative to torso), and flat dumbbell press certainly fit the bill. The use of free weights (versus machines) requires the greatest degree of neuromuscular coordination. As you move a completely unfixed object through space, you must support and control the weight in every direction. Machines, on the other hand, limit the ways in which the weight can be moved. By doing so, machines actually support the weight in certain directions, functionally increasing your strength in those directions. This explains why you can generally handle more pounds on a machine press, for example, than on a straight bench press.

When performing your work sets, remember to keep your chest out and your shoulders back or you will inadvertently use your trapezius muscles, cheating your pectorals of important mass-building stimulation. Begin by holding the weights roughly parallel to your chest. Exhale as you extend your arms upward, pushing the dumbbells toward the ceiling. At the top of the motion, bring the weights together for an isometric squeeze. Exhale during the concentric phase of the motion. Bring the dumbbells together for an isometric squeeze at the top of the motion. Inhale as you lower the weights slowly to a position where your elbows are either at or slightly below the surface of the bench and the dumbbells are at chest level.

🏠 Flyes

Primary movers: **Pectorals**

Flyes are a slightly more advanced movement that I don't recommend attempting until you have mastered the flat dumbbell press. With flyes, you start from a position of mechanical disadvantage. Hence, you will use a lighter weight than what you are accustomed to using for presses.

Lie on the bench with your arms extended out at the shoulder, elbows slightly bent, gripping the dumbbells with your palms facing

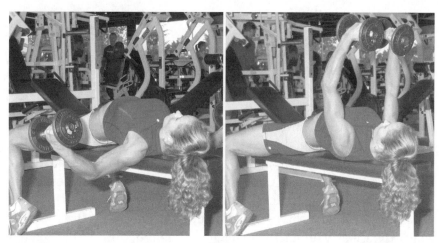

Flyes

up. Now, without changing the angle of your elbows, bring your arms together over your chest as if you were hugging a big tree trunk. Touch the dumbbells together at the top of the movement, then lower them slowly back to the starting position. Repeat to muscular fatigue.

Machine Press

Primary movers: **Pectorals**

When it comes to chest training, machines are a great way to go heavy with minimal injury risk. Many equipment lines offer a range of chest machines from decline (focusing on the lower pectorals) to steep incline (focusing on the upper pectorals and anterior shoulder). The latest equipment is designed to permit a variety of lifting angles with arm approximation at the peak of the excursion. If your gym doesn't include any such machines, maybe you should consider shopping for a new gym! If you commence your chest training using a machine, be sure to incorporate a warm-up set. Because your movements are somewhat restricted, it is more difficult, but not impossible, to cheat using a machine. To avoid cheating, always remember to keep your chest out and your shoulders back. The basic technique for the machine press is identical to that of the free-weight press described earlier. As with free weights, aim for three or four work sets in a low to moderate rep range.

🏠 Military Press

Primary movers: **Deltoids**

The military press is the mainstay of shoulder development. As is the case with the bench press, using dumbbells for the military press is not only more effective but also less stressful for the shallow gleno-humeral joint than using a barbell. As with any other upper body training, always maintain good posture when performing the movement. Keep your back straight, your chest out, and your gaze forward. It is helpful, though not absolutely essential, to utilize a short bench with an upright back support. Start by holding the weights at shoulder level, with your palms facing out. Exhale during the concentric phase as you push the weights straight up toward the ceiling. At the peak of the movement, bring the weights together for an isometric squeeze. Inhale as you slowly lower the weights back to the starting position.

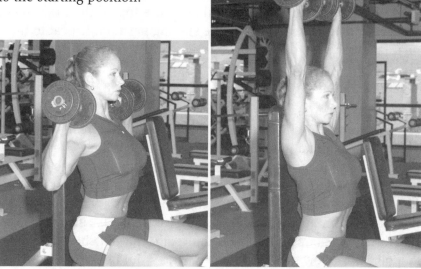

Military Press

🏠 Arnold Press

Primary movers: **Deltoids**

A variation of military press that I find extremely effective is known as the Arnold press, named after the guy who invented it, Mr.

Schwarzenegger himself. To correctly execute an Arnold press, start with two dumbbells held at shoulder height, palms facing toward you. As you press the weights up, exhale and gradually rotate your grip out. At the top of the movement, your palms should face out and away from your body. Slowly lower the weights as you inhale during the eccentric phase of the motion while simultaneously rotating your grip inward. Repeat until muscle fatigue.

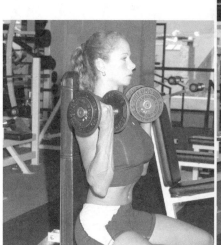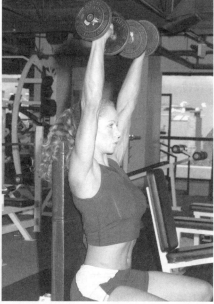

Arnold Press

🏠 Push-Ups

Primary movers: **Pectorals**

Push-ups work the pecs, delts, and triceps all at once, though the primary movers in standard push-ups are usually the pecs. Start with your hands flat on the floor, about shoulder width apart. With your arms extended to support your weight, keep your body straight, legs together, and toes firmly planted. Lower yourself in a steady, controlled manner until your chest brushes the floor, then return to the upright position. Do not let your back arch or your body sag at any point during the motion. Likewise, do not bend at the waist or let your weight rest on the floor between the decent and ascent. Perform each repetition with little or no pause in between, being sure to maintain muscular tension at all times. Three or four sets of push-ups should be performed to fatigue.

If regular push-ups are too difficult for you at this stage, try "girlie" push-ups, supporting yourself with your hands and, instead of your toes, your knees. Avoid bending at the waist. Your upper legs should stay aligned with your torso throughout the motion. If regular push-ups are not challenging enough, try decline push-ups, keeping your feet elevated on your training bench. As always, keep your back straight and do not bend at the waist.

PECTORAL DEFINING MOVEMENTS: ENHANCE YOUR CLEAVAGE LINE

The defining movements listed below target the inner fibers of your pectoral muscles, that is, the portion of your pectoral muscles that correspond to your cleavage line. In fact, working these fibers is just about the best way I know to naturally enhance your cleavage line and create the illusion of larger, firmer breasts.

Pec Deck

A great finishing exercise for inner pectorals is the pec deck. As with presses, you should be aware of your posture, keeping your chest out and shoulders back to resist using the trapezius muscles. At the start of the movement, extend your arms to either side of your body, with your elbows slightly bent. Exhale as you bring the machine's swing

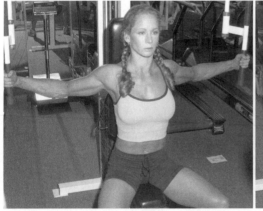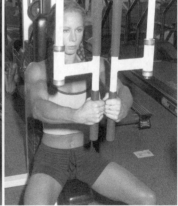

Pec Deck

arms toward the midline. The motion should feel as though you were hugging a barrel. Inhale as you slowly allow the arms to swing back to the start position.

Cable Flyes

Cable flyes are another tremendous finishing exercise. They can be accomplished with either a low-to-high (focusing on lower pectorals) or high-to-low (focusing on upper pectorals) motion, depending on where you attach the stirrups. As always, be aware of your form, keeping your chest out and your shoulders back. A high repetition range prevents cheating and helps hit the hard-to-reach muscle fibers that are called upon at the extremes of a motion range.

For an intense pump and a truly full range of motion, try performing cable flyes and the pec deck one arm at a time. Extend the excursion all the way across your body until your upper arm is mechanically blocked from further motion by your fully contracted chest muscles.

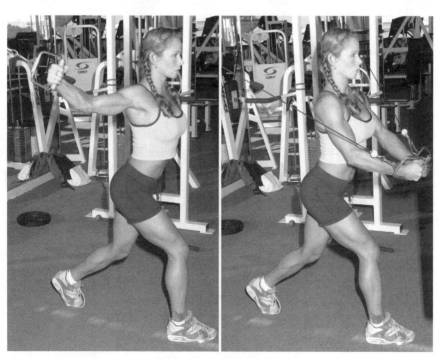

Cable Flyes—High-to-Low

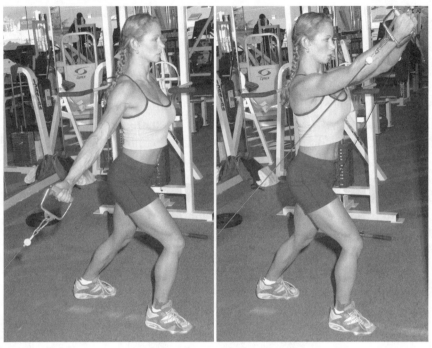

Cable Flyes—Low-to-High

REVIEW Tips for Building Spectacular Pectorals

1. The best exercises for the pectoral complex permit your arms to approach one another at the midline of the peak of the excursion.

2. Using dumbells, as opposed to a barbell, for presses is not only more effective but also less stressful for the shallow glenohumeral joint.

3. Remember to keep your chest out and your shoulders back or you will inadvertently cheat with your trapezius muscles.

4. Save exercises that target a specific portion of the pectoral complex, like the pec deck and cable flyes, for last.

DELTOID DEFINING MOVEMENTS: THREE GOOD HEADS PER SHOULDER

Round, defined deltoids are the crowning glory of a great physique. Because the deltoid complex is a relatively large muscle, it responds rapidly to weight training. However, utilizing proper technique when targeting your shoulders is critical to symmetrical development. Done correctly, shoulder training will improve your posture and make your waist appear slimmer. Done incorrectly, shoulder training will detract from good posture and induce a thick neck. To ensure good form and avoid this possibility, I recommend using the upper limits of the repetition ranges (10 to 15).

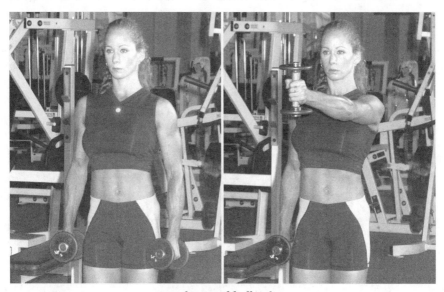 Anterior, Lateral, and Rear Deltoid Dumbbell Raises

When it comes to shoulder training, improper form is the number one pitfall for the overzealous novice who insists on using too much weight. Anterior (front), lateral (side), and posterior (rear) dumbbell raises should be accomplished with slow, even arcs. To begin, your feet should be roughly shoulder-width apart, with your knees slightly bent. Your chest should be out, shoulders back, and eyes straight ahead. For posterior raises, bend at the waist and knees as if you were about to dive into water. To be sure that your form is symmetrical, you may find it extremely helpful to face a mirror while performing deltoid raises. You may hold your arm at a slight angle to prevent locking at the elbow joint, but you should not flex or extend your lower arm during the motion. Likewise, do not use momentum

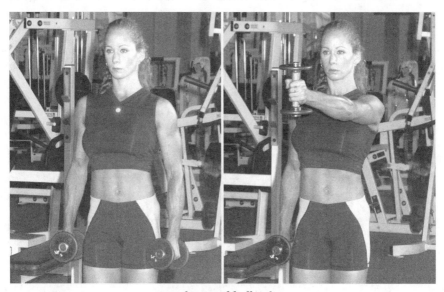

Anterior Dumbbell Raises

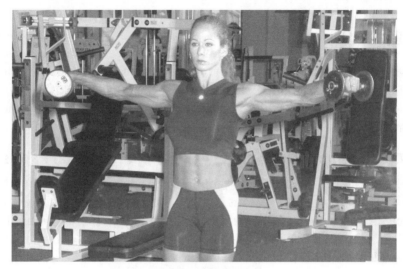

Lateral Dumbbell Raises

to raise the weight and do not bring your upper arms more than a couple inches above your shoulders at the peak of the excursion. (For these exercises, the deltoid muscle's range of motion is limited to below shoulder height; other muscles take over from there.)

As you perform deltoid raises, your rib cage expands. Hence, instead of following the traditional breathing rule (exhaling on the

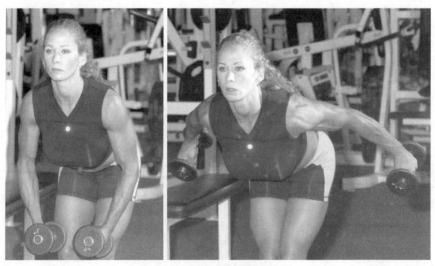

Rear Deltoid Dumbbell Raises

concentric phase and inhaling on the eccentric phase), implement the opposite breathing pattern: Inhale as you bring the weights up, and exhale as you steadily lower your arms to the starting position.

If you find that you are "shrugging" your shoulders at the peak, you are either using too much weight or you are doing too many repetitions. Once the shoulders start to shrug, it is a safe bet that you are cheating with the trapezius muscles. (Overly developed "traps," as they're affectionately known, will give you a neck like a football player, and unless you play football, you will probably want to avoid this eventuality.)

Don't forget what you can't see! The biggest mistake people make when training the deltoid complex is to neglect the rear portion of the muscle. This oversight paves the way for muscular imbalance, poor posture, and ultimately injury. Unfortunately, because it is so rarely used in our day-to-day existence, the rear deltoid is one of the most difficult muscles to isolate. It's very easy to cheat with the trapezius when working the rear deltoid. Be certain you feel the muscular contraction in your rear shoulder, not your neck. If you are having difficulty feeling rear shoulder raises in your rear deltoids, rather than leaning over to perform the movement, try lying on an incline bench.

Reverse Pec Deck

Try sitting backward on the pec deck for a reverse pec deck, a great exercise for rear deltoids. It may help to have a personal trainer or your training partner put light pressure over the posterior division to help you target the fibers. Because the rear deltoids often work in

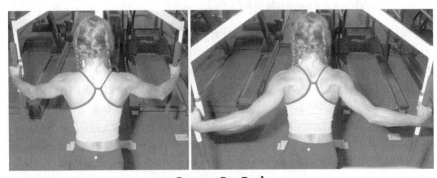

Reverse Pec Deck

conjunction with back muscles, I recommend training them on back day rather than shoulder day.

REVIEW Tips for Building Defined Delts

1. To avoid cheating with the trapezius muscles, always stand (or sit) with your chest out and shoulders back when performing exercises that target the anterior or lateral deltoid.

2. In order to reap the full benefits of shoulder work, isolate all three heads of the deltoid muscle with at least two sets of division-specific exercises.

3. For added endurance, try working the rear deltoids on back day rather than shoulder day.

TRICEPS POWER MOVEMENTS: SAY *NO* TO SAGGY UNDERARMS!

Contrary to popular belief, your triceps, not your biceps, compose the majority of the muscle found in your upper arm. Toned triceps are the antithesis of the dreaded "saggy underarm syndrome" that sends chills to the very core of so many women. Prevent (or reverse) this inevitability by building full, firm triceps.

Due to its scapular insertion, the posterior head of the triceps complex is best worked by exercises in which your arm remains superior to (higher than) your shoulder. This includes exercises for which you are lying down. In any triceps exercise, the shoulder should not rotate during the excursion. All movement should originate from the elbow joint.

Overhead Dumbbell Extensions

To minimize the risk of back injury, overhead extensions are best performed while seated. Start with the elbow bent to about 90 degrees and the upper arm held roughly perpendicular to the floor. Keeping the shoulder absolutely stable throughout the excursion, exhale as you straighten your arm at the elbow to bring the dumbbell directly overhead. Your triceps will experience maximal resistance during the excursion, as they contract. Slowly inhale as you return to the original position. Always control the weight to avoid both head and shoulder joint injury.

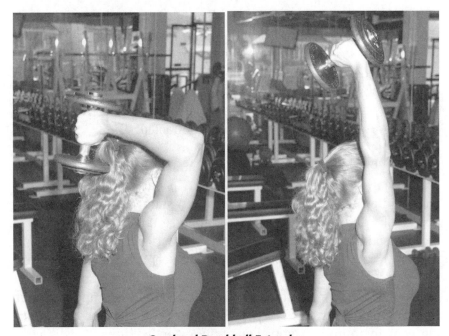

Overhead Dumbbell Extension

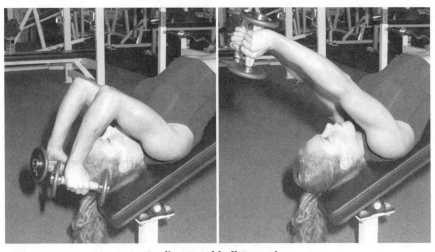 Decline Dumbbell Extensions

When executed correctly, decline extensions are among the most difficult and rewarding exercises. With conventional overheads, the

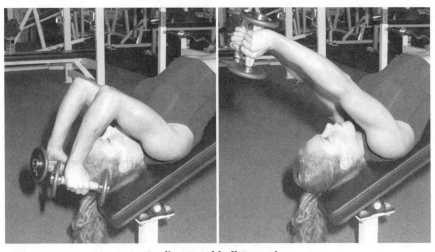

Decline Dumbbell Extension

arm is perpendicular to the floor at the top of the motion. Supporting the weight directly overhead with your elbow locked requires more balance than strength. Decline extensions are performed lying on a decline bench with your elbows positioned by your ears. At the top of the motion, your arms are fully extended but are not perpendicular to the gravity. Hence the triceps experience maximal resistance at the peak of the excursion, when fully contracted.

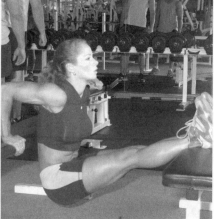 Bench Dips

Traditional dips are performed using two parallel bars and body weight. Because they tend to put your shoulder in an unstable degree of external rotation, I do not endorse this exercise. Instead, I recommend bench dips. At the start of your triceps training, you will probably want to use a single bench and keep your feet planted on the floor. To begin, sit on the edge of the bench. Place your hands on the bench on either side of your butt. Extend your legs and rest your heels on the floor in front of you. Slide your butt off the bench, holding your torso upright with your fully extended arms. This is your starting position. Now, inhale as you flex your elbows and lower your butt toward the floor. This is the eccentric phase of the motion. Descend until your upper arm is roughly parallel to the ground. For the concentric phase of the exercise, extend your elbows to push yourself back to the starting position.

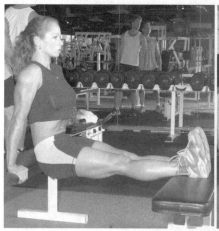 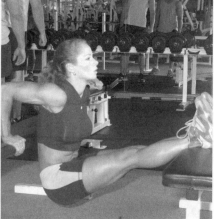

Bench Dips

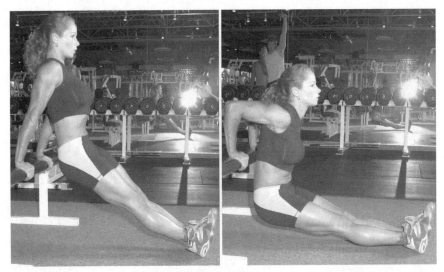

Easy Dips

For added challenge, try doing dips between two benches. One bench is used to support your arms, while the other is used to support the heels of your fully extended legs.

TRICEPS DEFINING MOVEMENTS: HONING THE HORSESHOE

Triceps defining movements are a wonderful way hone the horseshoe, so to speak. If you are striving for shape in addition to tone, the many variations of cable push-downs are a marvelous way to help bring out the anterior head of the triceps. To preferentially isolate the posterior head without involving multiple joints, nothing beats kick-backs.

Cable Push-Downs

Unlike extensions and kick-backs, cable push-downs place more emphasis on the anterior head of the triceps complex, and a well-defined anterior triceps is a sight to behold! Because this head is smaller than the posterior head, I suggest using lighter weight and doing push-downs as a finishing exercise, after the posterior head has been fatigued by power movements.

For conventional push-downs, begin by standing with your feet shoulder-width apart. Grasp the bar attachment with an overhand (palms down) grip. Bend your elbows to 90 degrees and angle your

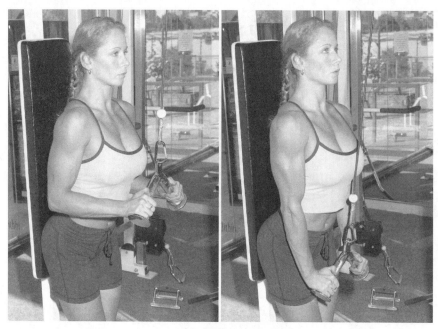

Cable Push-Downs

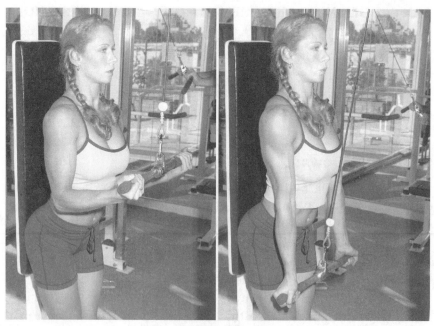

Reverse Cable Push-Downs

upper arms slightly forward (away from your body). By holding your arms slightly forward, the bar's progress during the concentric phase of the motion will not be impeded by your thighs. Likewise, the triceps will meet continued resistance at the bottom of the motion provided your fully extended arms are not quite perpendicular to the ground.

With your upper arms angled slightly forward, 90 degrees of elbow flexion places your hands slightly higher than your elbows at the start position. As you push the weight downward, virtually all movement should arise from the elbow joints. Your shoulders should remain stable during the full excursion. Pause at the bottom for an isometric squeeze before returning to the starting position.

When using the rope attachment for cable push-downs, I recommend pushing both down and out as you perform the movement. This will force your forearms to pronate as they extend at the elbow joints. Be sure to pause at the bottom of the motion for a half-count isometric squeeze. If you have access to a bar attachment that rotates, try using a reverse or underhand (palms up) grip to really feel the triceps contracting at the bottom of the movement.

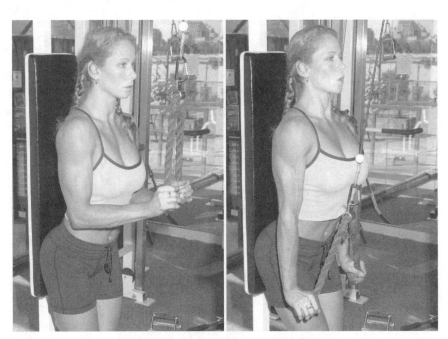

Cable Push-Downs with Rope Attachment

🏠 Kick-Backs

Kick-backs are a great way to incorporate pronation into your finishing exercises. You will need a low, flat bench. Begin by kneeling to the rear of the bench on your left knee. Plant your right foot firmly on the ground and place your left hand on the bench, supporting your upper body. Grip a dumbbell with your right hand, positioning your right arm at your side with your upper arm roughly parallel to your torso. For the starting position, your elbow should be bent at a 90 degree angle. Now, without moving your shoulder or upper arm, extend your forearm, from the elbow, out behind you. As you extend, remember to simultaneously rotate your grip outward and pronate your forearm. For proper form it's very important that your upper arm and shoulder remain stationary, so that all motion originates from your elbow and forearm. After a brief isometric squeeze at the top of the motion, slowly lower your forearm back to the starting position. Keep your back straight and your gaze forward as you repeat the exercise to muscular fatigue. When you've completed your work sets, switch sides and duplicate the exercise with your left arm.

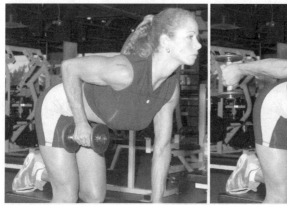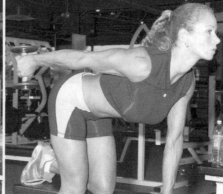

Kick-Backs

REVIEW Tips for Building Terrific Triceps

1. In order to work the full range of motion of the triceps, you must both extend your elbow and pronate your forearm. Incorporate at least one such movement each time you train triceps.

2. Multijoint power movements like extensions and bench dips emphasize the posterior head, or the bulk of the triceps complex.

3. In order to target the anterior head of the triceps, try finishing exercises like push-downs after the posterior head has been fatigued by power movements.

Considering Breast Augmentation Surgery?

How we see ourselves has enormous bearing on how others see us. To a large degree, our life's accomplishments are intimately linked to self-image. Looks play an undeniably pivotal role in our self-image, and community opinion flavors our individual perceptions of what "looks good." Lamentably, social trends are cruel dictators that do not often comply with nature or even good health. Over the past three decades, breast augmentation surgery has provided a means to increased self-esteem and confidence for tens of thousands of women who perceived themselves as underendowed. For women in entertainment (including the booming fitness industry) who depend on their looks to make a living, breast augmentation has become more than just a vanity issue.

If you are considering breast surgery for personal or professional reasons, realize that cosmetic enhancement does not have the power to transform fundamentally unhappy people into intoxicatingly fulfilled individuals. It probably won't change your intrinsic attitudes about life. But if you have spent years agonizing while you padded your bras, if you are painfully self-conscious or embarrassed, if your self-esteem is suffering as a result of your small chest size, getting a "boob job" could have a very real and positive impact on your life. To be honest, I know very few women who have undergone the procedure and regret it. Most say they would do it again in a heartbeat!

The decision to undergo the procedure is not a choice to be made lightly. The better advised you are about the potential risks, benefits, and results of the surgery, the better equipped you will be to make an intelligent, informed decision. The following is a list of the most commonly asked questions and answers surrounding breast augmentation.

What are the implants filled with?

In the United States, silicone gel-filled implants are currently unavailable to first-time augmentation candidates. Saline-filled implants are the established alternative. Both implant types utilize a pliable envelope made from silicone rubber. Most would agree that the silicone gel-filled implants feel more natural than their saline counterparts because the gel's consistency is closer to that of natural breast tissue. In addition, the silicone gel-filled implants are less likely to "ripple" when placed over the muscle. Lean individuals with over-the-muscle placement of saline-filled implants often develop slight rippling in the implant bag, which can be visible through the skin.

Are there different types of silicone envelopes?

The silicone envelope itself is available with either a rough or smooth texture. The nontextured implant bag is less likely to cause rippling; however, it increases the risk of capsular contracture, the most common complication of breast augmentation surgery. The development of a fibrous capsule around the implant is the body's normal response to the introduction of a foreign material. In 15 to 20 percent of augmentations, the fibrous capsule develops excess scar tissue and contracts around the implant, causing the breast to feel hard and rigid. The condition can be treated with surgical stripping of the capsule. In a small percentage of cases, capsular contracture will recur.

What's all the hype about silicone? Does it really cause autoimmune disease in some women?

According to two dozen studies involving thousands of women, there is absolutely no scientific data to support this concern.

What are the different surgical approaches to breast augmentation?

There are three primary surgical approaches for implant surgery: transaxillary (through the armpit), periareolar (under the nipple), and inframammary (through the skin fold beneath the breast). The periareolar incision provides the best aesthetic results. The healed scar is extremely well concealed compared to the other sites, and the results of implant placement are the best. You may have heard of a fourth approach through the umbilicus (belly button). Many surgeons eschew this method because proper placement of the implant through the navel is nearly impossible. Transumbilical implant surgery may also damage the inframammary fold, an anatomical violation that compromises the structural integrity of the breast and will likely lead to aesthetic deformities down the road.

Does going under the nipple increase the chances of lost sensation?

The risk of loss of sensation in the nipple or breast increases with increasing implant size and has nothing to do with surgical approach.

What about breast-feeding?

It is unlikely that implant surgery will interfere with breast-feeding.

What are the different implant placements?

There are two traditional implant placements: over the pectoralis muscle and under the pectoralis muscle. Neither approach is perfect. Placement over the pectoralis muscle increases the risk of capsular contracture, rippling, and drooping and is aesthetically less desirable especially in lean women. The submuscular placement, however, results in implant movement during exertion and can interfere with activities requiring use of the pectoralis muscle.

Partial coverage, in which only the upper portion of the implant lies beneath the pectoral muscle, is an innovative new approach that combines the best aspects of both placements. This procedure decreases the risk of capsular contracture, rippling, and drooping and is aesthetically very natural looking. At the same time, it causes minimal interference with pectoralis muscle function. In my opinion, partial coverage is the best placement for active women.

How long after undergoing the procedure do I have to take it easy?

Most women are able to resume normal daily activities, such as driving, within a few days following surgery. It is advisable to lay off all physical training including cardiovascular activities for two to three weeks in order to decrease the risk of complications. Weight lifting may be resumed gradually after this time with the avoidance of painful movements. A longer hiatus may be necessary before returning to heavy chest training.

What other risks should I know about?

As with any surgery, there is always the slight risk of infection, bleeding, delayed wound healing, and anesthesia complications. Your doctor will explain these risks to you in greater detail and will inform you if you are at an increased risk for specific complications.

What about mammograms? Will my doctor have a harder time reading them?

Women who have never undergone breast surgery normally have four different radiographs taken during a mammogram. Women who have had breast augmentation have an additional image taken. This is known as an Eklund Test and confers similar efficacy in detecting a cancerous tumor as standard mammography.

How much does the surgery cost?

Breast augmentation surgery generally runs between $4,000 and $10,000, though I have heard quotes as low as $2,500. Beware: you might get what you pay for. Conversely, a high price does not necessarily mean that a particular surgeon is the best.

How do I choose a doctor? Can any surgeon perform the operation?

Only a plastic surgeon is qualified to perform breast augmentation surgery. In the United States, a plastic surgeon must complete both a general and a plastic surgery residency, which entails a minimum of six years of postgraduate training (ten years, if you count medical school). During the course of residency, surgeons will observe, assist, and perform thousands of procedures. Their training is nothing short of exhaustive, and any board-certified plastic surgeon should be well qualified to perform implant surgery. Nevertheless, you should choose your surgeon wisely. Get more than one opinion. Research your doctor: collect references; ask to see his or her "book" of before and after pictures. Does he or she specialize in breast surgery? Is he or she board certified? You owe it to yourself to find out!

Awesome Abdominals

I s it wrong to covet chiseled abs? Only if you take offense at the capacity to attract the opposite sex in droves, radiate energy and passion for life, and enjoy a long and healthy existence. Exaggeration? Hardly! The lifestyle necessary to attain a body that warrants immortalization in marble transcends superficial vanity. Like it or not, it's virtually impossible to sculpt a six pack without doing an awful lot of things that are good for you.

Don't rush out and order the latest contraption you saw on the infomercial featuring Mr. Muscle, Ms. Figure, and Dr. Expert. Although ab machines can certainly help to strengthen your abs, there will be no chiseling of definition until you've taken the prerequisite steps to overall fitness. You see, all the crunches, sit-ups, and hanging leg raises in the world won't give you an etched midsection unless your body fat is already quite low. The single most effective means for shedding unwanted pounds is the consistent participation in cardiovascular exercise. See Chapter 8 for details.

FUNCTIONAL ANATOMY OF THE RECTUS ABDOMINUS AND OBLIQUES

Although abdominal training is not a terribly complicated venture, certain aspects deserve mention. The largest of the abdominal muscles is the rectus abdominus, a.k.a. the "six pack." The rectus abdominus acts to stabilize the trunk and flex the spine, bringing the rib cage and pelvis toward one another. The external obliques, located to either side of the rectus abdominus, are referred to as opposite-side rotators. The left side external obliques facilitate the movement

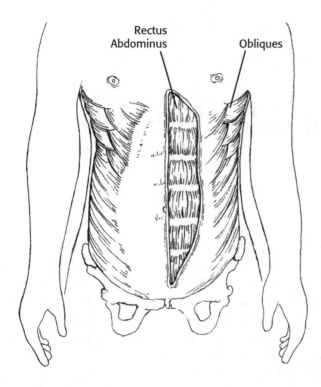

Rectus
Abdominus

Obliques

**The stomach,
showing the
rectus abdominus
and the obliques.**

of twisting your trunk to the right, and vice versa. The internal obliques lie beneath the external obliques and are configured so that their fibers actually run at right angles to the external obliques. As a result, they are same-side rotators.

The goal of abdominal training is to maximize the contribution of these three muscle groups while minimizing the involvement of hip flexors and spinal muscles. Surprisingly, some very traditional movements—including sit-ups, crunches beyond a 30-degree angle, supine leg raises, and rapid or weighted lateral flexion (side bends)—don't conform to these objectives. These exercises not only are inefficient for six-pack sculpting but can actually cause neck strain, back pain, and muscular imbalances.

In designing your abdominal program, make an effort to select movements that include both spinal flexion and rotation. For best results, hit your abs two to three times per week. Like any other body part, abdominal muscles adapt rapidly to new stimuli. To avoid tedium and ensure continued progress, frequently vary your workouts. Before you know it, you'll be sporting that six pack outside your belly.

BUNCHES OF CRUNCHES

Whether you're a rank beginner or seasoned veteran, floor exercises are a convenient and effective way to train your whole abdominal complex.

🏠 Basic Crunches

Basic crunches, which target the entire rectus abdominus, are the mainstay of abdominal development. Start by lying on your back with your knees bent and your feet flat on the floor. (Use a mat or carpeted area for comfort.) Refrain from the temptation to interlock your fingers behind your head. Instead, place your hands by your ears with your elbows pointed out. Then, without flexing your neck, contract your abdominal muscles and exhale as you bring your shoulder blades just off the floor. Hold the contraction for a half count at the peak of the motion, then inhale as you return to the starting position. Do three to four sets to the point of muscular fatigue.

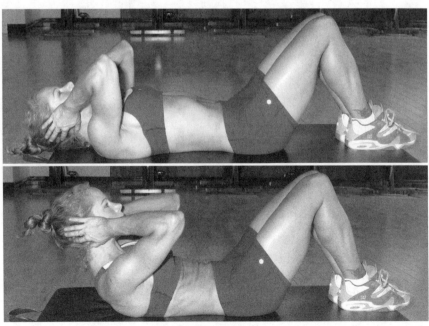

Basic Crunches

🏠 Side Crunches

By allowing your legs to fall to one side, you can easily modify basic crunches to target your oblique muscles with side crunches. As before, hold your hands by your ears and exhale as you contract to bring your shoulder blades off the floor. Hold the contraction for a half count at the top and inhale as you return to the starting position. Once muscular fatigue sets in, rest for 30 seconds, then let your legs fall to the opposite side and repeat.

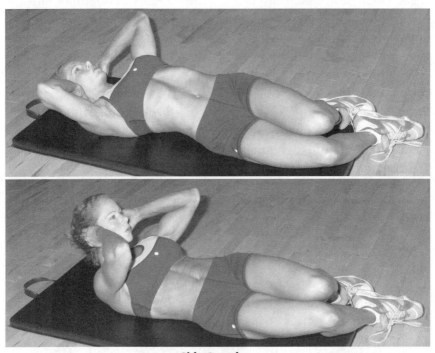

Side Crunches

🏠 Lying Hip Raises

Lying hip raises are a great exercise for hitting the lower abdominal muscles. Start by lying flat on the floor with your arms down at your sides. Point your legs straight up into the air so that they form a 90-degree angle with your torso. Keeping your head and shoulder blades flat on the mat, exhale as you contract your abdominal muscles and raise your hips off the floor. Tilt your pelvis toward your

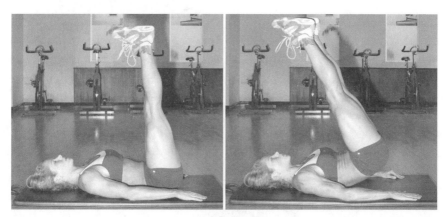

Lying Hip Raises

belly button, hold for a half count, and lower your hips back to the starting position. Repeat until muscular fatigue sets in.

Hanging Leg Raises

Hanging leg raises are a challenging way to target the entire abdominal complex, and they yield unbeatable results. Leg raises can be performed while hanging from arm slings, gripping a bar, or using a

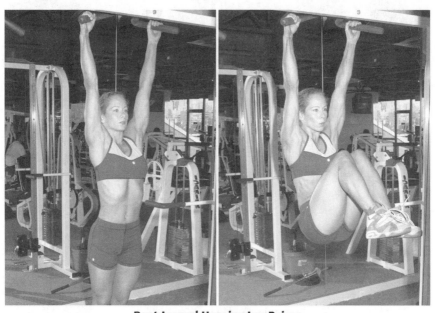

Bent-Legged Hanging Leg Raises

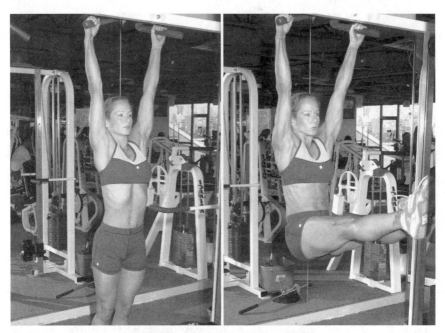

Straight-Legged Hanging Leg Raises

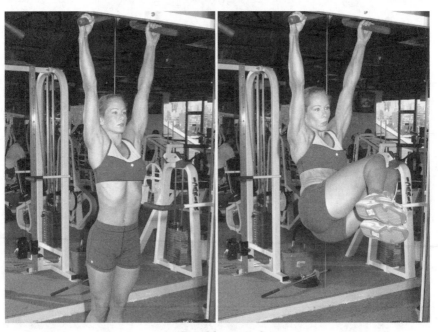

Hanging Side Leg Raises

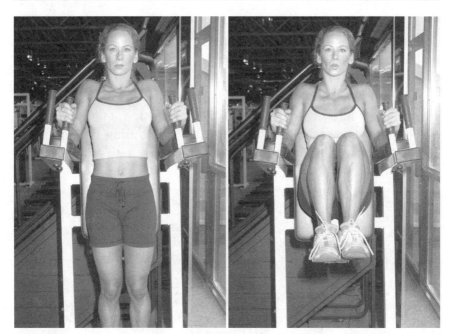

Hanging Leg Raises on Roman Chair

Roman chair. They can be accomplished with straight legs or bent knees. Simply raise your legs until your thighs are perpendicular to your torso, exhaling as you do so. For the eccentric phase of the motion, inhale while lowering your legs slowly and steadily to avoid "swinging" your entire body. Repeat until muscular fatigue prevents further repetitions.

The initial phase of the movement, as you raise your thighs to your torso, requires a majority contribution from your hip flexors, not your abdominal muscles. The portion of the motion with exclusively abdominal input begins as your thighs continue past 90 degrees to approach your torso.

Because it takes enormous strength and flexibility to bring your legs straight above your head, I recommend you start with bent-legged raises and gradually work your way up to straight-legged raises. Hanging side leg raises, generally performed with bent knees, are an excellent way to target the oblique muscles.

Cable Crunches

Cable crunches are a fabulous alternative to floor crunches for targeting the entire rectus abdominus. They can be performed standing or kneeling depending on your preference. Attach a rope to the upper pulley of a cable station and select an appropriate resistance. With your back to the machine, hold the rope ends firmly against your shoulders and contract your abdominal muscles. Exhale as you crunch. For the eccentric phase of the contraction, come up slowly and steadily, maintaining tension in the cable during the entire set. You should control the weight, and not the other way around.

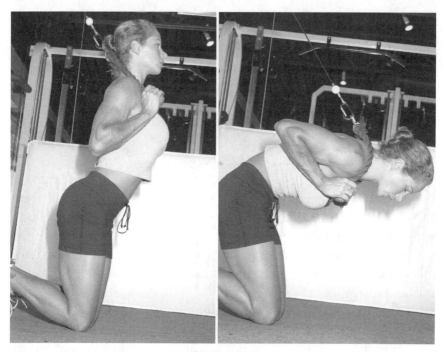

Cable Crunches

STAND UP AND STAY STRONG

Full-body strength training can greatly accelerate your quest for a six pack. Not only does it burn overall fat, but your increased muscularity will accelerate fat loss by making your body metabolically more active. In addition, strength training itself actually helps to chisel your emerging washboard. Virtually every movement in your weight-lifting repertoire calls for torso stabilization, which is accomplished primarily by your abdominals and low back muscles. The more exercises you perform while standing (versus sitting or lying), the greater the recruitment of abdominal and low back musculature, and the more quickly your abdominal muscles will be strengthened.

REVIEW Tips for Building Amazing Abs

1. Avoid sit-ups, crunches beyond 30 degrees (any more than just raising your shoulder blades off the floor), supine leg raises, and rapid or weighted lateral flexion (side bends).

2. Exhale during the concentric phase of the motion as you contract your abdominal muscles. Inhale during the eccentric phase.

3. Floor exercises are a convenient and effective way to train your abdominal muscles.

4. Hanging leg raises and basic crunches target the entire abdominal complex.

5. A full-body strength-training program will accelerate the development of a six-pack stomach.

6. Standing exercises targeting any muscle group will also build and strengthen both your abdominal and low back muscles.

Gorgeous Gams and Glutes

When I lived in California, Gold's Gym was the one place I could always go when the chips were down. The one place I knew I'd be treated right. Even in my darkest hour, I could show up with puffy eyes and a baseball cap pulled low to conceal as much of my blotchy face as possible. I'd wear an oversized sweat shirt with the fashion elegance of a horse blanket and a pair of black spandex tights applied sparingly over my rounded derriere and firm, shapely gams . . .

Yup. That was the whole key. The guys at the front desk would gush like lovesick puppies, falling over each other to compliment me on just how good I looked. Let's get real here. On those days, about the only thing separating me from my Neanderthal ancestors was a pair of opposable thumbs. But the guys loved my bottom half. And I loved that they loved it.

I'm lucky. My mother, who is pushing seventy, still has a perky butt and shapely thighs. And ten years of ice hockey and cycling have had an undeniably positive impact on my posterior contours, not to mention my thighs and calves. However, I maintain that everyone can build a butt and legs to be proud of. You simply need to arm yourself with effective movements, patience, and the drive to survive two days following intense training when it is too painful to rest your full weight on the toilet seat.

The Gluteal Complex

The gluteal complex is a combination of three distinct butt muscles:

FUNCTIONAL ANATOMY OF THE BUTT, THIGHS, AND CALVES

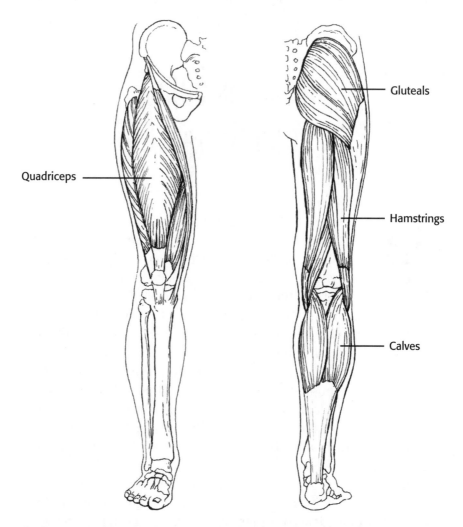

Quadriceps

Gluteals

Hamstrings

Calves

The front of the leg (left) showing the quadriceps muscle; and the back of the leg (right) showing the gluteal complex, hamstring, and calf muscle.

the gluteus maximus, gluteus minimus, and gluteus medius. The gluteus maximus is the largest muscle of the human body, and its primary function is to extend the hip and stabilize the hip joint. It is called into play when, for example, you are rising from a stooped position or climbing stairs. The gluteus medius and gluteus minimus are hip abductors. They are used when the leg is lifted to the side, such as when you push off during skiing or skating. Because of its large size, the gluteal complex responds best to relatively heavy weights.

The glutes, as they're called, work in close conjunction with both the hamstring and the quadricep muscles. In fact, all three major muscle groups contribute to multijoint power movements. Modifications in foot stance and/or machine angle allow you to shift the emphasis from behind your center of gravity (targeting primarily glutes and hamstrings) to in front of your center of gravity (targeting primarily quads). For symmetrical development, it is best to incorporate both approaches.

Hamstrings

The three muscles at the rear of the thigh are collectively referred to as the hamstrings. The proximal attachment of each hamstring is a protuberance known as the ischial tuberosity, a structure of the rear pelvis that supports your weight in the seated position. The three members of the hamstring complex are the semitendinous muscle, the semimembranous muscle, and the biceps femoris. Distally, the semitendinous and semimembranous muscles attach to the medial (inner) aspect of the rear of the tibia (shin bone). The biceps femoris inserts distally onto the back of the head of the fibula. The hamstrings work together to extend the hip and flex the knee.

Quadriceps

The quadriceps femoris, otherwise known as the quad, is composed of four separate heads. The rectus femoris is the largest single section. Its proximal attachment inserts onto different parts of the pelvis. The three minor heads, or vestiges, are the vastus lateralis, vastus medialis, and vastus intermedius, and they all attach proximally to the femur (thigh bone) and the connective tissue surrounding the femur. Distally, all four heads of the quadriceps femoris converge to form the quadriceps tendon, which surrounds and attaches to the patella (knee cap) before continuing on as the patellar ligament. The patellar ligament, in turn, attaches to the tibia. The quads work to both extend the knee and (via the rectus femoris) flex the hip.

Calves

The gastrocnemius muscle (calf muscle) has two heads, both of which attach to the femur. Distally, the two heads merge to form the tendo calcaneus (Achilles tendon). The gastrocnemius muscle acts to *plantar flex* the ankle, as when you stand on tiptoe.

SYNERGISTIC MULTIJOINT POWER MOVEMENTS

Many glute and thigh development aficionados live and die by the squat. Several variations exist: free squats, bench squats, Smith squats, and hack squats. They are all great ways to target your butt and thighs. Done improperly, however, squats can be extremely hard on the knees and low back, especially when handling poundages that really challenge the gluteal complex. To avoid injury, insist on good form. If you've never done squats before, start with a light weight.

During any squatting movement, be sure to keep your chin up, eyes raised, and back straight as you drop down to and rise from the

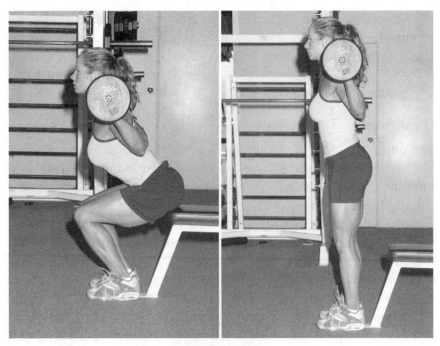

Bench Squats

squat. Inhale as you lower the weight and exhale as you ascend back to the starting position. (I recommend descending no further than the point at which your knees are angled at 90 degrees and your thighs are roughly parallel to the floor.) Beyond that, squats place enormous stress on the patellar tendon and internal structures of the knee joint. If you are a beginner doing free squats, I recommend that you use a bench to limit your descent.

Squats for Glutes and Hamstrings

To preferentially target glutes, squats should be done using a wide (roughly twice shoulder width), toes-out stance.

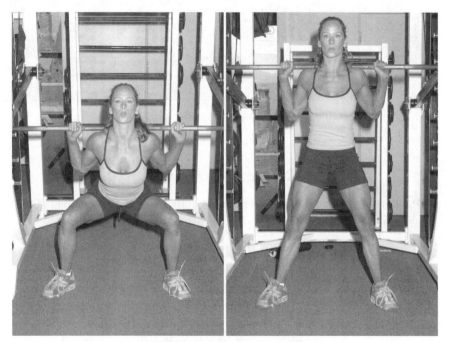

Squats for Glutes and Hamstrings

Squats for Quads

To preferentially target the quads, use a narrow (shoulder width), toes-straight stance. Because you will probably be able to handle considerably more weight using the glute/hamstring stance, always start lighter with the quad stance.

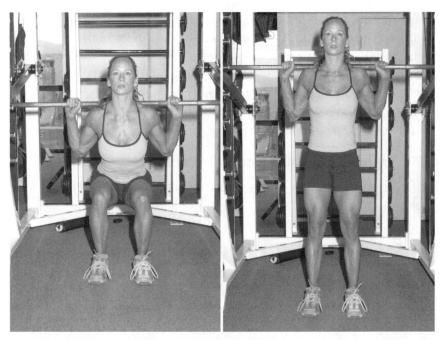

Squats for Quads

A Squat Is a Squat Is a Squat

There are several different types of squat. Although their setups differ, the fundamental motion for each is virtually the same.

- **Free squats** are performed from a freestanding position, without mechanical support.

- **Smith squats,** which also begin from a freestanding position, are performed using a "Smith machine" that employs a tracking device to eliminate the possibility of any side-to-side or twisting motion.

- **Hack squats** are performed on an apparatus that positions the user on an incline plane relative to the floor. Like Smith squats, hack squats use a tracking apparatus to limit free movement.

- **Bench squats,** a variation of the free squat or Smith squat, strategically place a bench behind the squater to limit the extent of the downward motion. They prevent the squatter's thighs from descending below the parallel so that the knees do not bend beyond 90 degrees.

Leg Press for Glutes and Hamstrings

I swear by the leg press. If the press is adjustable, push the seat forward to its fully upright position. By then placing your feet high on the stand, you create a relatively acute angle between thighs and upper body. From here, only a short range of motion is required to straighten the legs, and most of the power behind the movement originates in the gluteus maximus, not the quads.

Inhale as you lower the weight and exhale as you raise it back to the starting position. As with squats, keep the angle of your knee at or above 90 degrees to prevent undue strain on the patellar tendon and knee joint. Try executing half of your sets with a wide stance to really hit your gluteus maximus. For the rest, bring your feet together in order to maximize the contribution of gluteus medius and minimus.

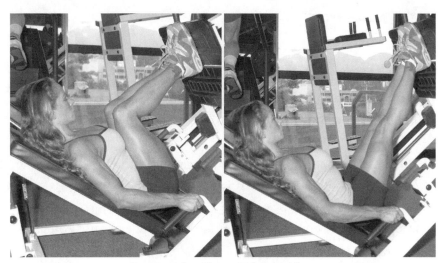

Leg Press for Glutes and Hamstrings

Leg Press for Quads

The leg press is also a tremendous exercise for targeting your quads. By simply positioning yourself differently, you can shift the emphasis from the rear to the front of your legs. First, you will use a much lighter weight than you used to train your glutes. Second, rather than adjusting the seat to create an acute angle between your torso and thighs, recline the seat back as far as it will go and place your feet low on the stand to create a relatively obtuse or wide angle between your thighs and upper body. You should find that you feel the exercise in your quads, not your glutes. Once again, I don't recommend allowing the angle of your knee to fall below 90 degrees, as this places enormous stress on the patellar tendon and knee joint.

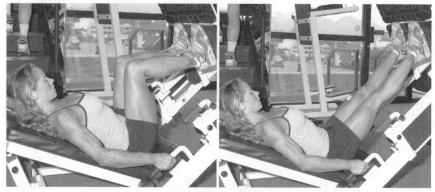

Leg Press for Quads

REVIEW Get the Most from Leg Training

1. The best exercises for toning and firming your legs and butt are multijoint power movements that flex and extend both the hip and knee.

2. When performing squats, avoid descending below a knee angle of 90 degrees to minimize the risk of knee injury.

3. For squats, use a wide, toes-out stance to target glutes and hamstrings and a narrow, toes-straight-ahead stance to target quads.

4. For the leg press, use an acute thigh-torso angle to best target glutes and hamstrings and an obtuse thigh-torso angle to best target quads.

GLUTE AND HAMSTRING DEFINING MOVEMENTS

If you want a really great rear view, a handful of muscle-specific defining movements will ensure that your butt and hamstrings are chiseled to perfection. Unlike the multijoint power movements described above, you do not need to use heavy weights to see results. Use a managable weight and strict form, including a pronounced isometric squeeze at the peak of the contraction.

🏠 Sissy Squats for Glutes and Hamstrings

Unlike traditional squats, sissy squats provide a great burn using nothing more than body weight. They should be done as a finishing movement, after you've completed heavy sets of leg presses or squats. You will require a fixed, sturdy item that can be gripped at waist height to support your weight. A stair banister, squat rack, or even a door knob will all serve the purpose. Grasp the object, then drop an imaginary line straight down from it and place your feet on either side of the point where the line meets the ground. Lean back, straightening your legs as you extend your arms. Your weight should be on your heels, and you'll be in a "water skiing" position. Keeping your back and arms straight, lower yourself to the point at which your butt nearly contacts the floor, then return slowly to the start position. Concentrate on tightening the butt as you come up, and hold an isometric squeeze for a two-count at the top of each repetition. With strict attention to form, it's difficult to exceed 30 reps per set.

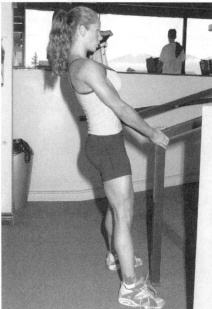
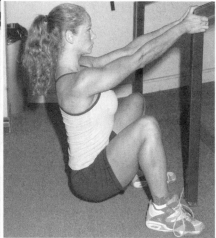

Sissy Squats

Abductor Machine

The abductor machine is another great finishing movement; it targets primarily the gluteus medius and minimus. The most important thing to remember here is to keep your back straight and hips and torso stationary as you move through the motion range.

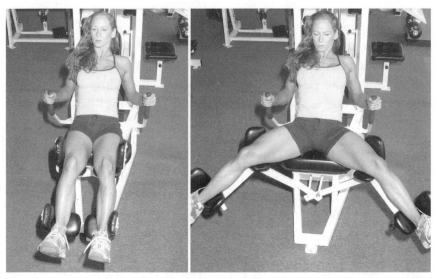

Abductor Machine

Prone Hamstring Curls

One of the best ways to accentuate your butt is to better define the tie-ins it shares with your hamstrings. I have rarely observed a physique with full, rounded hamstrings that was not crowned by an equally impressive butt. The two seem to go hand in hand. Prone hamstring curls are a marvelous way to build strong, defined hamstrings. They should be done slowly, with a fluid, controlled motion. An isometric squeeze at the height of the contraction, when your hamstrings are fully flexed against the weight, will accentuate the peak of the muscle.

I recommend avoiding heavy weights that would sacrifice form. Likewise, you should never jerk the weight up or cheat with momentum. Always keep your hips firmly planted against the pad. Butt-in-air spine arching signals cheating with the muscles of your lower back while they are in a vulnerable position of mechanical disadvantage. In other words, you're just begging for an injury. Hopefully your gym's prone hamstring curl machine is angled at the hips, a slight variation that does wonders for preventing back strain.

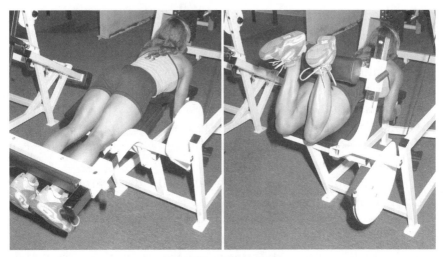

Prone Hamstring Curls

🏠 Straight-Legged Dead Lifts

In my humble opinion, straight-legged dead lifts are the single most effective exercise for working the butt and hamstring tie-ins. They are definitely not for anyone with a history of low back pain. Stand

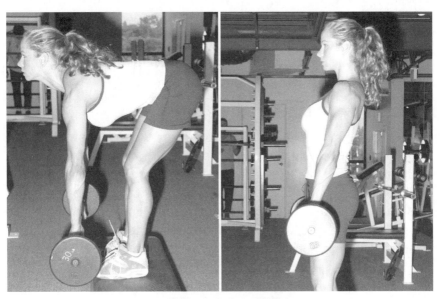

Straight-Legged Dead Lifts

on a raised platform, knees slightly bent, holding a barbell with a shoulder-width grip. Keeping your back very straight, bend forward at the hips. Depending on your strength and flexibility, the plates of the barbell might descend below the platform's surface. Never allow your back to arc forward. If you feel this happening, use less weight. Your knees should remain stationary and slightly bent throughout the range of motion. As you return to the starting position, concentrate on squeezing your butt. An isometric two-count at the top can really add to the burn.

When it comes to straight-legged dead lifts, I strongly advise training in a repetition range of at least 15 to 20, with strict attention to form to prevent back strain. If possible, take a jacuzzi or at least sit in a hot bath after your first encounter with this beast; even using a relatively light weight will probably make you wish you could pee standing up.

REVIEW Tips for Building Gorgeous Glutes and Smashing Hamstrings

1. During sissy squats, incorporate an isometric squeeze at the top of each repetition.

2. During prone leg curls, keep your hips firmly planted against the pad.

3. When performing straight-legged dead lifts, aim for a repetition range of at least 15 to 20 with strict attention to form to prevent back strain.

QUAD DEFINING MOVEMENTS

As you learned in Chapter 8, there is no way to target a problem area for fat burning. However, as you continue to implement a healthy, high-protein diet plus regular, moderate exercise, a new you will begin to emerge. The layer of subcutaneous fat covering your muscles will gradually melt away, revealing the firm, toned physique beneath. Soon, you will begin to discern the outline of muscle beneath your skin. Eventually, the actual separations between different muscular insertions will also become visible. The following exercises can significantly enhance this process, endowing you with sleek, athletic thighs.

Leg Extensions

Before commencing this exercise, be certain that the machine is adjusted to your height and the length of your lower leg. The foot pad should rest just above your ankle joint, so that you are able to point your toes toward the ceiling during the entire movement. Use a weight that challenges you but does not cause knee pain.

Whenever you do leg extensions, I recommend including at least one set targeting each of the three minor quad heads, or vestiges. To target the vastus lateralis (the muscle head that lies to the outside of your thigh), point your toes inward during the exercise. To target the vastus medialis (the muscle head that lies to the inside of your thigh), point your toes out. To target the vastus intermedialis (the centeral head that lies below the rectus femoris), point your toes up.

As always, perform the exercise in a steady, controlled manner. Hold the peak of the contraction (the point at which your legs are fully extended) for a half count. Do not relax after the concentric or active phase of the motion; instead, during eccentric phase, as you lower the weight, maintain tension. Repeat to muscular fatigue.

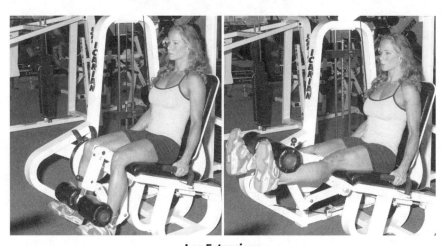

Leg Extensions

🏠 Sissy Squats for the Quads

Sissy squats for the quads are similar to sissy squats for the glutes and hamstrings (see page 231). However, instead of leaning back and "water skiing" as you did for glute training, keep your back aligned at a 90-degree angle to the floor. With your back straight, lower yourself to the point at which your butt nearly contacts the floor, then return slowly to the starting position. You should feel the movement in your quads, with minimal contribution from your butt.

Adductor Machine

If flabby inner thighs are your personal nightmare, you can tone and firm the muscles with an occasional visit to the adductor machine. Keep your back straight and your chest out when performing this exercise. For added pump, include a two-count isometric squeeze at the peak of each contraction.

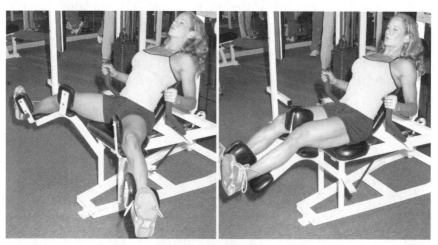

Adductor Machine

REVIEW Sculpting Quintessential Quads

1. Leg extensions are the best exercise for enhancing the strength of the individual quad muscles.

2. When you do leg extensions, include at least one set to target each of the three minor heads, or vestiges.

3. Sissy squats can be modified to create a quad-defining workout.

CARVE YOUR CALVES

Perhaps more than any muscle group, your calves' size and shape are influenced largely by genetic factors. I've seen couch potatoes with calves that would have looked far more appropriate on a world-class sprinter. By the same token, I've known professional body-builders who trained their calves relentlessly but never observed the sort of growth that characterized the rest of their bodies. Regardless of your genetic predisposition, you can build calves to be proud of.

Pound for pound, your calves are the strongest muscles in your body, and for good reason. Your calves are called into play whenever you bend your ankle or point your toe. They contract against the full weight of your body every time you walk, run, jump, or climb. Because they are capable of enormous feats of endurance, your calves may respond best to repetitive tasks such as stair climbing and cycling. If you are not happy with the progress your calves are making with your basic weight routine, incorporate a calf-intensive component to your cardiovascular training. Climbing stairs, climbing hills, or cycling are excellent ways to meet your aerobic requirements while giving your calves an added challenge.

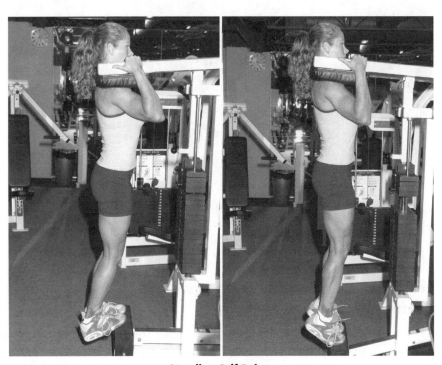

Standing Calf Raises

🏠 Calf Raises

The technique for doing calf raises (also known as calf extensions) is identical regardless of whether you perform them seated, standing, or lying within a hack squat apparatus. If your feet are flat on the floor or platform, simply extend your calves (by rising up on your toes) against the resistance as far as your flexibility allows. Return to the starting postion and repeat to fatigue. If you are on the edge of a step or platform, you can increase your motion range and stimulate additional muscle fibers by allowing your heel to descend below the step or platform during the eccentric phase of the contraction.

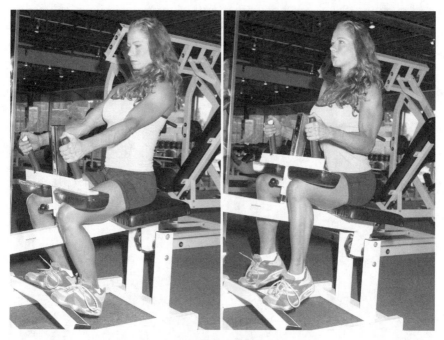

Seated Calf Raises

Leg Press, Sissy Squats, Smith Squats, Hack Squats, Seated and Standing Raises

My reasons for combining upper leg and calf training are more logistical than physiological. Because a number of quad exercises are amenable to calf training, it's simply convenient to train your calves

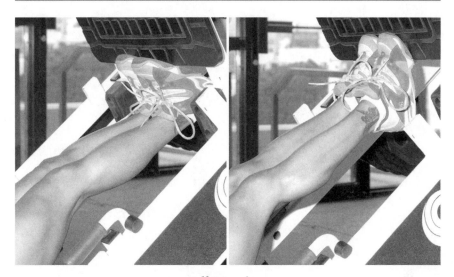

Calf Extensions

with your thighs and butt. For example, between sets of leg press, it's simple and timesaving to do a set of calf extensions on the leg press. You won't even have to get up from the machine. The same holds true for sissy squats (using body weight), Smith squats, and hack squats. If you don't manage to fulfill your calf-training requirements during your upper leg workout, add a few sets of machine calf raises. Alternate between seated and standing calf raises in order to stimulate the muscle from different angles and through varying motion ranges.

Appendices

Appendix A

Healthy Choice Food Lists

COMPLETE PROTEINS

Dietary recommendations: Have approximately one 100-calorie serving per meal. For more information, please refer to Chapter 3.

Dairy	100-Calorie Serving
Fat-free or low-fat cheeses	3–4 slices
Fat-free cottage cheese	5 oz.
Fat-free ricotta cheese	2.5 oz.
Fat-free yogurt	8 oz.
Skim milk	10 oz.
Eggs	**100-Calorie Serving**
Egg whites	6 large
Egg beaters	4 servings
Poultry	**100-Calorie Serving**
Chicken breast (skinless)	3 oz.
Cold cuts (low/non-fat)	3 oz.
Turkey breast	3 oz.
Turkey (ground, 93% fat free)	3 oz.
Red Meat	**100-Calorie Serving**
Beef (ground round)	2 oz.
Cold cuts (low/non-fat)	3 oz.
Flank	2 oz.
Lean cut steak	2 oz.

Round steak	2 oz.
Seafood	**100-Calorie Serving**
Abalone	4 oz.
Bass	4 oz.
Bluefish	3 oz.
Carp	3 oz.
Catfish	3.5 oz.
Clams	6 oz.
Cod	4.5 oz.
Crab	4 oz.
Crab meat (imitation)	3.5 oz.
Flounder	4.5 oz.
Grouper	4 oz.
Haddock	4.5 oz.
Halibut	3.5 oz.
Lobster	4 oz.
Monkfish	4.5 oz.
Mussels	4 oz.
Ocean pearch	3.5 oz.
Oysters	7 large
Oysters (canned)	4 oz.
Pike	4 oz.
Pollock	4 oz.
Red snapper	4 oz.
Shark	3 oz.
Shrimp	8 large
Sole	4.5 oz.
Squid	5 oz.
Swordfish steak	3.5 oz.
Trout	4 oz.
Tuna steak	2.5 oz.
Tuna white meat	$2/_3$ can
White fish	2.5 oz.

STARCHY CARBOHYDRATES AND SIMPLE SUGARS

Dietary recommendations: Have one or two 100-calorie servings per meal, depending on your body type, activity level, and weight-loss goals.

Breads and Cakes	100-Calorie Serving
Angel food cake	1½ oz.
Bagels	½ medium
Biscuit	1 medium
Bread sticks	9 small sticks
Bun (burger)	1 medium
Corn bread	1½ oz.
Dinner roll	2 medium
Doughnut	1 oz.
English muffin	½
French bread	1 oz.
Italian bread	1 oz.
Pancakes (oat bran)	2 small
Pancakes (buckwheat)	2 small
Pancakes (plain)	2 small
Pancakes (whole wheat)	1 medium
Pita bread	½
Pound cake	¾ oz.
Pumpernickel	1½ slices
Raisin bread	1 slice
Rye bread	1½ slices
Sourdough bread	1½ slices
Sponge cake	1 oz.
Taco shells	1 shell
Tortillas (low-fat or non-fat)	1 small
Waffles	1 medium
White bread (enriched)	1½ slices

Whole-wheat bread	1½ slices
Whole-wheat roll	2 medium
Cereals	**100-Calorie Serving**
General Mills Buc Wheats	¾ cup
General Mills Cheerios	1 cup
General Mills Kix	1½ cup
General Mills Total	1 cup
General Mills Wheaties	1 cup
Kellogg's All Bran	½ cup
Kellogg's Bran Buds	½ cup
Kellogg's Corn Flakes	1 cup
Kellogg's Corn Pops	1 cup
Kellogg's Product 19	¾ cup
Kellogg's Raisin Bran	¾ cup
Kellogg's Rice Krispies	1 cup
Kellogg's Special K	1 cup
Nabisco Cream of Wheat	2½ tablespoons (uncooked)
Post 40% Bran Flakes	⅔ cup
Post Grape Nuts	¼ cup
Post Grape Nut Flakes	1 cup
Post Oat Flakes	⅔ cup
Post Oat Meal	⅓ cup (uncooked)
Post Shredded Wheat (biscuit)	1 biscuit
Post Shredded Wheat (spoon size)	⅔ cup
Quaker Puffed Rice	2 cups
Quaker Puffed Wheat	2 cups
Ralston-Purina Bran Chex	⅔ cup
Ralston-Purina Corn Chex	1 cup
Ralston-Purina Rice Chex	1 cup
Fruit	**100-Calorie Serving**
Apple	2 small
Apple sauce (unsweetened)	1 cup

Apricot	6 small
Banana	1 medium
Blackberries	1 $\frac{1}{2}$ cups
Blueberries	1 cup
Boysenberries	1 cup
Cantaloupe	1 medium
Cherries	1 cup
Cranberries	2 cups
Currants	3 cups
Grapefruit	1 large
Grapes	1 cup
Kiwi	2 small
Mango	$\frac{1}{2}$ medium
Melon (honeydew)	1 medium
Nectarine	2 small
Orange	2 small
Papaya	1 medium
Passion fruit	2 medium
Peach	2 small
Pear	1 medium
Pineapple chunks	1 cup
Plum	4 medium
Raspberries	1 cup
Strawberries	2 cups
Tangerine	2 small
Watermelon	3 cups
Fruit Juice	**100-Calorie Serving**
Apple juice	7 oz.
Apricot juice	7 oz.
Grapefruit juice	6 oz.
Grape juice	6 oz.
Orange juice	7 oz.

Pineapple juice	6 oz.
Grains	**100-Calorie Serving**
Brown rice (uncooked)	1/6 cup
Corn (canned)	3/4 cup
Minute Rice (uncooked)	2/3 cup
Popcorn (air popped, no butter)	5 cups
White rice (uncooked)	1/6 cup
Legumes	**100-Calorie Serving**
Black beans (dry)	1 oz.
Brown beans (dry)	1 oz.
Fava beans (cooked)	4.5 oz.
Garbonzo beans (dry)	1 oz.
Kidney beans (cooked)	3.3 oz.
Lima beans (canned)	4 oz.
Navy beans (cooked)	4 oz.
Pinto beans (dry)	1 oz.
Red beans (cooked)	3.3 oz.
Refried beans (fat-free, canned)	4 oz.
Soybeans (cooked)	4 oz.
Pasta (cooked)	**100-Calorie Serving**
Fettuccini	1/2 cup
Vermicelli	1/3 cup
Spaghetti	1/2 cup
Spaghetti (protein enriched)	1/2 cup
Spinach pasta	1/2 cup
White pasta	2/3 cup
Wheat pasta	1/2 cup
Root Vegetables	**100-Calorie Serving**
Beets	8 oz.
Carrots	14 oz.
Parsnips	6 oz.

Potatoes (baked)	4 oz.
Potatoes (boiled)	5 oz.
Sweet potato (baked)	3 oz.
Rutabaga	10 oz.
Yam	4 oz.

FIBROUS CARBOHYDRATES

Dietary recommendation: Enjoy all you can eat.

Alfalfa sprouts	Celery	Lettuce
Artichokes	Collard greens	Mushrooms
Asparagus	Cucumber	Okra
Bamboo shoots	Dandelion greens	Onion
Bean sprouts	Eggplant	Peas
Broccoli	Endive	Pea pods
Brussels sprouts	Green beans	Peppers
Cabbage	Kale	Spinach
Cauliflower	Lentil sprouts	Squash

HEALTHY FATS

Dietary recommendations: If fats comprise less than 20 to 25 percent of your total caloric intake, supplement at each meal with the appropriate amounts of these healthy fats.

Fat	100-Calorie Reference Serving Size
Avocado	2 oz. or $\frac{1}{4}$ medium
Calavo oil	1 tablespoon
Fish oil	1 tablespoon
Flaxseed oil	1 tablespoon
Hemp oil	1 tablespoon
Olive oil	1 tablespoon
Peanut butter	1 tablespoon
Soybean oil	1 tablespoon

Appendix B

Glycemic Index of Common Carbohydrates

Foods with a glycemic index of more than 60 are considered to fall high on the glycemic scale.

HIGH-GLYCEMIC-INDEX (HGI) STARCHY CARBS	
Breads and Cakes	**Glycemic Index**
Angel food cake	67
Bagels	72
Bread stuffing	74
Bun (burger)	87
Corn bread	63
Croissant	67
Dinner roll	71
French bread	95
Italian bread	95
Kaiser roll	73
Melba toast	70
Rye bread	64
Taco shells	68
Waffle	76
White bread	71
Whole-wheat bread	68
Whole-wheat roll	68

Cereals	Glycemic Index
General Mills Cheerios	74
Ralston-Purina Corn Chex	83
Kellogg's Corn Flakes	83
Nabisco Cream of Wheat	70
Post Grape Nuts	68
Post Oat Flakes	80
Quaker Puffed Wheat	74
Kellogg's Raisin Bran	80
Ralston-Purina Rice Chex	89
Kellogg's Rice Krispies	82
Post Shredded Wheat	69
General Mills Total	76
Fruit	
Cantaloupe	65
Pineapple	66
Watermelon	72
Fruit Juice	
Pineapple	66
Pasta	
Gnocchi	67
Rice pasta	92
Legumes	
Fava beans	79
Root Vegetables	
Beets	64
Parsnips	97
Potato (baked)	85
Potatoes (boiled, mashed)	73

LOW-GLYCEMIC-INDEX (LGI) STARCHY CARBS	
Breads	**Glycemic Index**
Bulgur bread	53
Linseed rye bread	55
Pita bread	57
Pumpernickel	50
Whole grain bread	48
Cereals	
Kellogg's All Bran	42
Kellogg's Bran Buds	53
Ralston-Purina Bran Chex	58
Muesli	56
Oatmeal	49
Kellogg's Special K	54
Fruits	
Apple	38
Apricot	31
Banana	54
Cherries	22
Grapefruit	25
Grapes	46
Kiwi	53
Mango	54
Orange	44
Peach	42
Pear	37
Plum	39
Fruit Juice	
Apple juice	58
Grapefruit juice	48
Orange juice	52

Grains	Glycemic Index
Brown rice	55
Popcorn	55
Sweet corn	55
White rice	58
Legumes	
Black beans	30
Brown beans	38
Garbonzo beans	33
Kidney beans	29
Lima beans	46
Navy beans	38
Pinto beans	39
Red beans	29
Soybeans	18
Pasta	
Fettuccini	46
Vermicelli	50
Spaghetti	37
Spaghetti (protein enriched)	37
White pasta	41
Root Vegetables	
Carrots (cooked)	39
Sweet potato	54
Yams	51

Appendix C
Exercise Routines

FULL-BODY ROUTINES

Routine A requires two 25- to 30-minute sessions per week and works all your major muscle groups. After a week or two, you may wish to move on to routine B, which increases the intensity with additional sets. This routine requires two weekly sessions of about 45 minutes. Of course, if you are satisfied with the progress you are making with routine A, you should feel free to stick with it indefinitely.

Full-Body Routine A

Session length: 25 to 35 minutes

Recommended schedule: Train two or three times a week.

Rest between sets: 30 to 45 seconds

Muscle Group	Sets	Reps
Abdominals	3–4	20–30
Back	3–4	15–20
Biceps		
power movements	2–3	15–20
Calves	2–3	15–20
Hamstrings/Glutes		
power movements	2–3	15–20
Pectorals		
power movements	2–3	15–20

Muscle Group	Sets	Reps
Quads		
power movements	2–3	15–20
Shoulders		
power movements	2–3	15–20
Triceps		
power movements	2–3	15–20

Full-Body Routine B

Session length: 45 to 60 minutes
Recommended schedule: Train two or three times a week.
Rest between sets: 30 to 45 seconds

Muscle Group	Sets	Reps
Abdominals	3–4	20–30
Back	3–4	15–20
Biceps		
power movements	3–4	15–20
Calves	3–4	15–20
Hamstrings/Glutes		
power movements	3–4	15–20
Pectorals		
power movements	3–4	15–20
Quads		
power movements	3–4	15–20
Shoulders		
power movements	3–4	15–20
lateral delts	2–3	15–20
Triceps		
power movements	3–4	15–20

SPLIT ROUTINES

Two-Day Split Routine A

Session length: 25 to 35 minutes

Recommended schedule: Train two or three days a week, alternating zones.

Rest between sets: 45 to 60 seconds

DAY 1: UPPER BODY ZONE		
Muscle Group	**Sets**	**Reps**
Back	4–6	12–15
Biceps power movements	2–3	12–15
Pectorals power movements	3–4	12–15
Shoulders power movements	3–4	12–15
Triceps power movements	2–3	12–15

DAY 2: LOWER BODY ZONE		
Muscle Group	**Sets**	**Reps**
Abdominals	3–4	20–30
Hamstrings/Glutes power movements	3–4	12–15
Quads power movements	3–4	12–15
Calves	3–4	12–15

Two-Day Split Routine B

Session length: 45 to 60 minutes

Recommended schedule: Train two or three days a week, alternating zones.

Rest between sets: 45 to 60 seconds.

DAY 1: UPPER BODY ZONE		
Muscle Group	**Sets**	**Reps**
Back	4–6	12–15
Biceps power movements	3–4	12–15

Pectorals

power movements	4–6	12–15
defining movements	2–3	12–15

Shoulders

power movements	4–6	12–15
lateral deltoids	2–3	12–15

Triceps

power movements	3–4	12–15

DAY 2: LOWER BODY ZONE		
Muscle Group	**Sets**	**Reps**
Abdominals	3–4	20–30
Hamstrings/Glutes		
power movements	4–6	12–15
defining movements	3–4	12–15
Quads		
power movements	4–6	12–15
defining movements	3–4	12–15
Calves	4–6	12–15

Three-Day Split Routine A

Session length: 25 to 35 minutes

Recommended schedule: Train three times a week, alternating zones.

Rest between sets: 60 to 90 seconds

DAY 1: EXTENSOR ZONE		
Muscle Group	**Sets**	**Reps**
Abdominals	3–4	15–20
Pectorals		
power movements	3–4	6–10
defining movements	2–3	10–15
Shoulders		
power movements	3–4	6–10

lateral delts	2–3	10–15
Triceps		
power movements	3–4	6–10

DAY 2: LOWER BODY ZONE		
Muscle Group	**Sets**	**Reps**
Calves	3–4	8–12
Hamstrings/Glutes		
power movements	4–6	6–10
defining movements	2–3	10–15
Quads		
power movements	4–6	6–10
defining movements	2–3	10–15

DAY 3: FLEXOR ZONE		
Muscle Group	**Sets**	**Reps**
Abdominals	3–4	15–20
Back	6–8	8–12
Biceps		
power movements	3–4	6–10
defining movements	2–3	10–15

Three-Day Split Routine B

Session length: 45 to 60 minutes

Recommended schedule: Train three times a week, alternating zones.

Rest between sets: 60 to 90 seconds

DAY 1: EXTENSOR ZONE		
Muscle Group	**Sets**	**Reps**
Pectorals		
power movements	6–8	6–10
defining movements	3–4	10–15

Shoulders

power movements	6–8	6–10
lateral delts	3	10–15
medial delts	3	10–15

Triceps

power movements	3–4	6–10
defining movements	3–4	10–15

DAY 2: LOWER BODY ZONE		
Muscle Group	**Sets**	**Reps**
Hamstrings/Glutes		
power movements	6–8	6–10
defining movements	3–4	10–15
Quads		
power movements	6–8	6–10
defining movements	3–4	10–15
Calves	6–8	6–15

DAY 3: FLEXOR ZONE		
Muscle Group	**Sets**	**Reps**
Back	8–12	8–12
Biceps		
power movements	3–4	6–10
defining movements	3–4	10–15
Shoulders		
rear delts	3–4	10–15
Abdominals	4–6	12–15

Four-Day Power Split Routine

Session length: 45 to 60 minutes

Recommended schedule: Train four times per ten days, alternating zones.

Rest between sets: 2 to 4 minutes

DAY 1: EXTENSOR ZONE		
Muscle Group	**Sets**	**Reps**
Pectorals		
power movements	9–12	3–8
Triceps		
power movements	9–12	3–8

DAY 2: LOWER EXTENSOR ZONE		
Muscle Group	**Sets**	**Reps**
Quads		
power movements	9–12	3–8
Calves	9–12	3–8
Abdominals	3–4	8–12

DAY 3: FLEXOR ZONE		
Muscle Group	**Sets**	**Reps**
Back	12–16	5–10
Biceps		
power movements	6–8	3–8

DAY 4: MIXED ZONE		
Muscle Group	**Sets**	**Reps**
Hamstrings/Glutes		
power movements	9–12	3–8
Shoulders		
power movements	9–12	3–8
Abdominals	3–4	8–12

CIRCUIT TRAINING

Full-Body Circuit-Training Routine

Session length: 25 to 35 minutes
Recommended schedule: Train two or three times a week.
Rest between exercises: 0 to 5 seconds
Repetitions per set: 15 to 30

Perform one set of a multijoint power *or* defining movement for each of the following muscle groups:

- Quads
- Calves
- Glutes/Hamstrings
- Chest
- Back
- Shoulders
- Biceps
- Triceps
- Abdominals

Repeat 2 or 3 times.

Two-Day Split Circuit-Training Routine B

Session length: 25 to 35 minutes
Recommended schedule: Train two or three times a week, alternating zones.
Rest between exercises: 0 to 5 seconds
Repetitions per set: 15 to 30

Day 1: Upper Body Zone

Perform one set of a multijoint power *or* defining movement for each of the following muscle groups:

- Chest
- Back
- Shoulders
- Biceps
- Triceps

Repeat 4 times.

Day 2: Lower Body Zone

Perform one set of a multijoint power *or* defining movement for each of the following muscle groups:

- Quads
- Calves
- Glutes/Hamstrings
- Abdominals

Repeat 4 times.

Three-Day Split Circuit-Training Routine

Session length: 25–35 minutes.

Recommended schedule: Train three times a week, alternating zones.

Rest between exercises: 0 to 5 seconds

Repetitions per set: 15 to 30

Day 1: Upper Body Pull Zone

Perform one set of multijoint power movements (during each of the first three circuits) followed by one set of defining movements (during each of the last three circuits) for each of the following muscle groups:

- Back
- Biceps
- Rear deltoids
- Abdominals

Repeat 6 times.

Day 2: Lower Body Zone

Perform one set of a multijoint power *or* defining movement for each of the following muscle groups (Use two different exercises per body part):

- Quads
- Calves
- Glutes/Hamstrings

Repeat 6 to 8 times.

Day 3: Upper Body Push Zone

Perform one set of a multijoint power *or* defining movement for each of the following muscle groups:

- Chest
- Triceps
- Abdominals
- Shoulders (but not the rear deltoids)

Repeat 6 times.

Appendix D

Exercises for Specific Muscle Groups

An asterisk (*) indicates an exercise that may be performed at home.

ABDOMINALS

- Cable crunches
- Crunches*
- Hanging leg raises*
- Lying hip raises*
- Side crunches*
- Roman Chair

BACK

- Bent-over barbell rows*
- Bent-over dumbell rows*
- Cable rows
- Lat cable pull-downs
- T-bar rows
- Wide-grip chin-ups*

BICEPS

Power Movements

- Alternating dumbell curls*
- Barbell curls*
- Preacher curls

Defining Movements

- Concentration curls*
- Overhead cable curls

CALVES

- Hack squat
- Leg press
- Seated calf raises*
- Sissy squat*
- Smith squat
- Standing calf raises*

GLUTES/HAMSTRINGS

Power Movements

- Bench squats*
- Free squats*
- Hack squats
- Leg press
- Smith squats

Gluteal Defining Movements

- Abductor machine
- Sissy squats*

Hamstring Defining Movements

- Prone leg curls
- Straight-legged dead lifts*

PECTORALS

Power Movements

- Decline bench press*
- Flat dumbell press
- Flyes*
- Incline dumbell press*
- Machine press*
- Push-ups*

Defining Movements

- Cable flyes
- Pec deck

QUADRICEPS

Power Movements

- Bench squats*
- Free squats*
- Hack squats
- Leg press
- Smith squats

Defining Movements

- Adductor machine

- Leg extensions
- Sissy squats*

SHOULDERS

Power Movements

- Arnold press*
- Military press*

Anterior Deltoid Defining Movements

- Front dumbell raises*

Lateral Deltoid Defining Movements

- Lateral dumbell raises*

Posterior Deltoid Defining Movements

- Bent-over dumbell raises*
- Reverse pec deck

TRICEPS

Power Movements

- Overhead dumbell extensions*
- Decline dumbell extensions*
- Bench dips*

Defining Movements

- Cable push-downs
- Rope push-downs
- Reverse push-downs
- Kick-backs*

Index

About the Author

Christine Lydon, M.D., completed her undergraduate training at Brown University, where she majored in neurobiology and French literature. She went on to attend the Yale University School of Medicine, where she became one of the most published medical students in the country. During her third year, Dr. Lydon was honored with the prestigious Howard Hughes Research Award for her work in the area of sports medicine. After graduating in 1994, Dr. Lydon chose to apply her medical training and research background to the sports fitness industry.

Since then, Dr. Lydon has worked as an independent consultant for several of the largest sports nutrition companies in the world and designed the diet protocol used at an award-winning Los Angeles health club chain. Dr. Lydon also acted as the personal fitness consultant to numerous Hollywood celebrities, including supermodel Carre Otis, comedian Richard Pryor, and writer/director Quentin Tarantino.

Dr. Lydon doesn't limit her involvement with the health industry to consulting for corporations and celebrities. Her years as a journalist and scientific writer for popular magazines like *Martial Arts Training, Powerlifting USA, Martial Arts Illustrated, Men's Fitness, Oxygen, MuscleMag International, Physical,* and *American Health and Fitness* have earned Dr. Lydon an enormous following among fitness enthusiasts and elite athletes alike. She is widely regarded as one of the premier women's fitness writers of North America. Dr. Lydon is also one of the most photographed physique models in the world. She has appeared in dozens of leading health periodicals, including *Muscle* & *Fitness, MuscleMag, Ironman, Natural Bodybuilding, Oxygen,* and *Planet Muscle,* and was the cover model for the inaugural issue of Playboy's *Hardbodies.*

Having the unlikely combination of medical training and celebrity as a fitness model provides Dr. Lydon with a unique perspective of the fitness industry. Readers place their confidence in Dr. Lydon's commentaries because, as her photos clearly illustrate, she practices what she preaches.